Review of Gynecologic and Breast Pathology

Review of Gynecologic and Breast Pathology

Ivan Damjanov MD PhD
Professor
Department of Pathology
The University of Kansas School of Medicine
Kansas City, Kansas, USA

Semir Vranic MD PhD
Assistant Professor
Department of Pathology
Clinical Center and School of Medicine, University of Sarajevo
Sarajevo, Bosnia and Herzegovina

Faruk Skenderi MD MSc
Senior Teaching Assistant
Department of Pathology
Clinical Center and Faculty of Health Sciences, University of Sarajevo
Sarajevo, Bosnia and Herzegovina

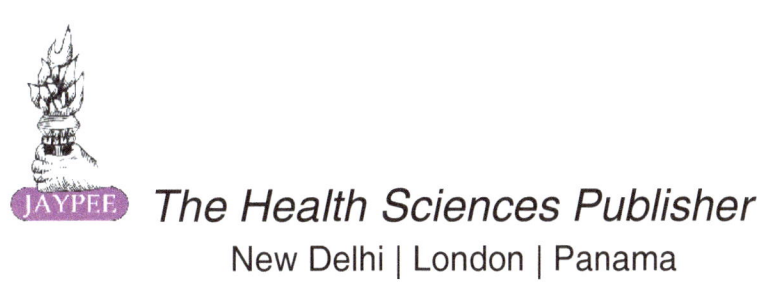

JAYPEE *The Health Sciences Publisher*
New Delhi | London | Panama

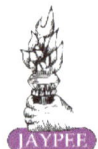 **Jaypee Brothers Medical Publishers (P) Ltd**

Headquarters

Jaypee Brothers Medical Publishers (P) Ltd
4838/24, Ansari Road, Daryaganj
New Delhi 110 002, India
Phone: +91-11-43574357
Fax: +91-11-43574314
Email: jaypee@jaypeebrothers.com

Overseas Offices

J.P. Medical Ltd
83 Victoria Street, London
SW1H 0HW (UK)
Phone: +44 20 3170 8910
Fax: +44 (0)20 3008 6180
Email: info@jpmedpub.com

Jaypee Brothers Medical Publishers (P) Ltd
17/1-B Babar Road, Block-B, Shaymali
Mohammadpur, Dhaka-1207
Bangladesh
Phone: +08801912003485
Email: jaypeedhaka@gmail.com

Jaypee-Highlights Medical Publishers Inc
City of Knowledge, Bld. 235, 2nd Floor,
Clayton, Panama City, Panama
Phone: +1 507-301-0496
Fax: +1 507-301-0499
Email: cservice@jphmedical.com

Jaypee Brothers Medical Publishers (P) Ltd
Bhotahity, Kathmandu, Nepal
Phone: +977-9741283608
Email: kathmandu@jaypeebrothers.com

Website: www.jaypeebrothers.com
Website: www.jaypeedigital.com

© 2017, Jaypee Brothers Medical Publishers

The views and opinions expressed in this book are solely those of the original contributor(s)/author(s) and do not necessarily represent those of editor(s) of the book.

All rights reserved. No part of this publication may be reproduced, stored or transmitted in any form or by any means, electronic, mechanical, photocopying, recording or otherwise, without the prior permission in writing of the publishers.

All brand names and product names used in this book are trade names, service marks, trademarks or registered trademarks of their respective owners. The publisher is not associated with any product or vendor mentioned in this book.

Medical knowledge and practice change constantly. This book is designed to provide accurate, authoritative information about the subject matter in question. However, readers are advised to check the most current information available on procedures included and check information from the manufacturer of each product to be administered, to verify the recommended dose, formula, method and duration of administration, adverse effects and contraindications. It is the responsibility of the practitioner to take all appropriate safety precautions. Neither the publisher nor the author(s)/editor(s) assume any liability for any injury and/or damage to persons or property arising from or related to use of material in this book.

This book is sold on the understanding that the publisher is not engaged in providing professional medical services. If such advice or services are required, the services of a competent medical professional should be sought.

Every effort has been made where necessary to contact holders of copyright to obtain permission to reproduce copyright material. If any have been inadvertently overlooked, the publisher will be pleased to make the necessary arrangements at the first opportunity.

Inquiries for bulk sales may be solicited at: jaypee@jaypeebrothers.com

Review of Gynecologic and Breast Pathology

First Edition: **2017**

ISBN: 978-93-5270-047-9

Printed at

Preface

This book of questions and answers deals with common and not so common pathologic entities encountered in the female genital organs and the breast. We have written this book primarily for pathologists and their trainees and suggest that it can be used as a review text, for continuing medical education (CME), a study guide, or as ancillary material during their studies of major textbooks. However, we also hope that it might be used by senior students, trainees in gynecology, surgery or oncology, and even as a CME book by their attendings.

We envisioned the book primarily as a brief review for specialists or advanced trainees who have a solid background in pathology. The book contains over 350 questions and we estimate that a serious student could finish it in 5 to 10 hours. However, the book could be used in many other ways. For example, for those who prefer to study a certain topic by first reading the questions, this compilation of questions and brief answers could serve as an introduction to further studies from more comprehensive and voluminous gynecologic pathology or breast pathology textbooks. The textbooks that we have used as reference points and also for possible further studies are listed of the end of this book. Some readers could also use our book as a source of key words and common abbreviations, and even less common data that can be found only in recent publications. Such data are usually from journals referenced next to the answers, included typically for more demanding readers who want to pursue the problem even further. For teachers of pathology and gynecology, the books could serve as a source of test questions and topics for discussions and seminars.

Most of the questions and answers are textual, but some questions are based on microphotographs of important pathologic entities. Accordingly, we have included in the book over 115 color microphotographs including immunohistochemical and in situ hybridization images.

In addition to basic pathology of the vulva, vagina, cervix, endometrium and myometrium, fallopian tubes, ovary, placenta and trophoblastic tumor, as well as breast pathology, at the end of the book we have included a separate chapter on immunohistochemistry and molecular biology/cytogenetics of tumors in these organs. For readers who are pathologists, such data are already essential components of their diagnostic workload. For gynecologists, surgeons and oncologists, these topics are becoming more and more important because in many instances new genetic data may critically direct the modalities of treatment of their patients. For some of our clinical colleagues, this chapter might be a good review; and for those less experienced in modern applied molecular and cell biology, these data might be a stimulus for further studies. Your impressions, comments and critical remarks may be sent to us by email to:semir.vranic@gmail.com.

Ivan Damjanov
Semir Vranic
Faruk Skenderi

Contents

Chapter 1   Vulva, Vagina and Cervix   1

Chapter 2   Uterus   24

Chapter 3   Fallopian Tubes   55

Chapter 4   Ovary   64

Chapter 5   Placenta   113

Chapter 6   Breast   129

Chapter 7   Immunohistochemistry and Genetics   168

Bibliography   *185*

Abbreviations

ACC	–	Adenoid cystic carcinoma
ADH	–	Atypical ductal hyperplasia
AFP (αFP)	–	Alpha fetoprotein, serum protein found in fetal and neonatal blood. It is normally secreted by yolk sac cells and fetal liver cells; also secreted by yolk sac tumors in mixed germ cell tumors or yolk sac carcinoma, and hepatocellular carcinoma.
ALDH1	–	Aldehyde dehydrogenase 1, a protein preferentially expressed in endometrioid carcinomas of the ovary.
AR	–	Androgen receptor
β-hCG	–	Beta human chorionic gonadotropin, normally secreted by trophoblastic cells; also secreted by gestational and nongestational choriocarcinoma or choriocarcinoma cells in mixed germ cell tumors.
BMT	–	Borderline mucinous tumor of the ovary
BRCA genes	–	Include *BRCA1* and *BRCA2* tumor suppressor genes that are involved in repair of damaged DNA. Germline mutations of both genes are responsible for the majority of familial breast and ovarian cancers.
BST	–	Borderline serous tumor of the ovary
CHM	–	Complete hydatidiform mole
CHEK2	–	Checkpoint kinase 2; it is a tumor suppressor gene, involved in signaling processes related to DNA damage.
CD	–	Cluster of differentiation, a designation followed by a specific numbers, given to group of proteins used as markers for lymphoid and hematopoietic cells and the molecular biologic/immunohistochemical classification of lymphomas and several other tumors.
CDH1	–	E-cadherin gene, encoding a cell adhesion molecule that is typically mutated in lobular breast cancer and diffuse gastric cancer. Germline mutations of *CDH1* gene cause familial cancer syndrome called hereditary diffuse gastric cancer (HDGC).
CDKN1	–	Cyclin-dependent kinase inhibitor 1C, a protein encoded by the maternally imprinted *CDKN1C* gene. Also known as p57^{kip2}.
CEP17	–	Chromosome 17 centromere; its probe is usually used by in-situ hybridization assays (Fluorescent or chromogenic/FISH/CISH) to evaluate the *HER-2/neu* gene copy number in patients with breast cancer (*HER2/CEP17* ratio).
CHM	–	Complete hydatiform mole
cKIT	–	Receptor tyrosine kinase encoded by *KIT* gene, a proto-oncogene discovered as human equivalent of viral oncogene *v-kit*. It is also known as stem cell growth factor receptor (SCFR) or tyrosine-protein kinase kit.
CMV	–	Cytomegalovirus
CTNNB1	–	β-catenin gene that is essential part of the WNT signaling pathway. It is mutated in desmoid tumors (fibromatosis) as well as in a subset of colorectal, thyroid, liver, ovarian, endometrial and skin cancers.
DCIS	–	Ductal carcinoma in situ
D2.40 (podoplanin)	–	Marker of lymphatic endothelium, but also expressed in dysgerminoma
DICER	–	A highly conserved enzyme belonging to the RNase III family of nucleases that specifically cleave double-stranded RNAs, and removes toxic RNAs.

EMA	–	Epithelial membrane antigen; EMA is glycoprotein on cell surface and is expressed by most glandular and ductal epithelial cells.
ER	–	Estrogen receptor
ESS	–	Endometrial stromal sarcoma, a tumor composed of cells that resemble endometrial stromal cells.
FEA	–	Flat epithelial atypia
FOXL2	–	A forkhead transcription factor with a DNA binding domain. It plays a critical role in the development of the ovary. *FOXL2* gene is mutated in over 90% of all adult granulosa cell tumors, and is thus considered to be important for the pathogenesis of these tumors.
FSH	–	Follicle-stimulating hormone
GCDFP-15	–	Gross cystic disease fluid protein 15
HELLP	–	Syndrome including hemolysis, elevated liver enzymes, low platelet count.
HER-2/neu	–	Human epidermal growth factor receptor 2; a member of the family of epidermal growth factor receptors; amplified in ~15–20% of all breast cancers.
HGSC	–	High-grade serous carcinoma of the ovary
HIV	–	Human immunodeficiency virus
HM	–	Hydatidiform mole
HMG1 and 2	–	High mobility group of nuclear non-histone proteins containing HMG-box domain, expressed in leiomyomas
HNPCC	–	Hereditary nonpolyposis colorectal carcinoma
HPV	–	Human papillomavirus
HSV	–	Herpes simplex virus
IHC	–	Immunohistochemistry
ISH	–	In situ hybridization assay including fluorescent (FISH) or chromogenic (CISH) techniques.
JGCT	–	Juvenile granulosa cell tumor
JAZF1/SUZ12	–	Fusion gene of JAZF1, acronym for Juxtaposed with another zinc finger gene, and *SUZ12* (suppressor of zeste-12 protein). Typically found in 50% high-grade endometrial stromal sarcomas.
Ki-67	–	A protein that is encoded by the *MKI67* gene. A sensitive marker of proliferation. Ki-67 has diagnostic and prognostic utility in many cancers. Other markers that are used for the evaluation of tumor cell proliferation include proliferating cell nuclear antigen (PCNA), topoisomerase IIα (Topo2α), and phosphohistone H3 (PPH3).
KRAS	–	Oncogene, human equivalent of Kirsten Rous sarcoma virus (*v-ras*)
LCIS	–	Lobular carcinoma in situ
LH	–	Luteinizing hormone
MALT	–	Mucosa-associated lymphoid tissue lymphoma
MED12	–	A subunit of the multiprotein complex mediator, an evolutionary-conserved regulator of transcription, mutated in most uterine leiomyomas and mammary fibroadenomas.
MGA	–	Microglandular adenosis
MLH1	–	MutL homolog 1 gene inactivated in hereditary nonpolyposis colorectal carcinoma and 10% endometrioid carcinoma of the uterus caused by this germline mutation
MYB	–	A gene, which is a member of the MYB family of transcription factors.
NCB	–	Needle core biopsy
NFIB	–	Nuclear factor 1 B-type
NGS	–	Next-generation sequencing assay, a new high-throughput technique, which may sequence thousands or millions of sequences in one reaction.
NLRP7	–	NACHT, leucine rich repeat, and PYD containing protein 7, a gene mutated in hereditary hydatidiform mole.
NOS	–	Not otherwise specified
OHSS	–	Ovarian hyperstimulation syndrome
p16	–	Cyclin-dependent kinase 2A inhibitor p16^{INK4}, a protein encoded by tumor suppressor gene *CDKN2A* gene; it is used in IHC for the diagnosis of cervical intraepithelial neoplasia.
p53	–	Protein encoded by *TP53* tumor suppressor gene. It is the most commonly mutated gene across the all cancer subtypes. Germline mutations of the *TP53* gene cause Li-Fraumeni syndrome.

p63	–	Protein encoded by the gene of the same name, belonging to the *TP53* gene family. It is involved in the stratification of squamous epithelium (positive in basal and parabasal cell of normal squamous epithelium) and a marker for myoepithelial cells; a good IHC marker for differentiating intraepithelial and invasive squamous carcinoma, but expressed in other tumors as well.
p57^{kip2}	–	Officially known as CDKN1 (cyclin-dependent kinase inhibitor 1C), a protein encoded by the maternal imprinted *CDKN1C* gene.
pCR	–	Pathologic complete response; related to the evaluation of the breast cancer patients treated with neoadjuvant (preoperative) chemotherapy. There are many evaluation tools of which MD Anderson Residual Burden calculator (RBC) has been shown to have the best reproducibility.
PASH	–	Pseudoangiomatous stromal hyperplasia.
PAX	–	Paired-box containing genes, which play important roles in the development and proliferation of multiple cell lines and development of several organs. Antibodies to *PAX2* and *PAX8* have a diagnostic utility in histopathologic diagnosis of tumors.
PEComa	–	Perivascular epithelioid cell tumor. It is a family of mesenchymal neoplasms composed of perivascular epithelioid cells. The neoplastic cells are typically positive for melanocytic and myogenic markers.
PHM	–	Partial hydatidiform mole
PIK3CA	–	Phosphatidylinositol-4,5-bisphosphate 3-kinase catalytic subunit alpha; *PIK3CA* is involved in various cell processes including cell proliferation and death and represents *one of the most commonly* mutated and amplified genes across the cancers.
PNET	–	Primitive neuroectodermal tumor
POC	–	Product of conception
POF	–	Premature ovarian failure
PCOS	–	Polycystic ovary syndrome
PR	–	Progesterone receptor
PTCH1	–	Protein patched homolog 1, the member of the patched family.
PTEN	–	Phosphatase and tensin homolog gene, which encodes the phosphatase and tensin protein, inactivated by mutation or deleted in most endometrioid endometrial carcinomas of the uterus and ovary; germline mutations of the *PTEN* gene cause Cowden syndrome that predisposes to multiple hamartomas and an increased risk of certain cancers (breast cancer, thyroid cancer, and endometrial cancer).
SALL4	–	Sal-like protein 4, a transcription factor encoded by a member of the *Spalt-like* (*SALL*) gene family, *SALL4* also known as key embryonic stem cells factor.
SBT	–	Serous borderline tumor of the ovary
SCOUT	–	Secretory cell outgrowths, also known as benign epithelial hyperplasia. They consists of hyperplastic foci composed of secretory cells, which may be ciliated, or show pseudostratification resembling endometrial epithelium, and are p53 negative.
SET	–	Solid endometrioid transitional pattern of high-grade serous carcinoma often found in women with germline BRCA mutations.
SIN	–	Salpingitis isthmica nodosa
SLCT	–	Sertoli-Leydig cell tumor of the ovary
SMA	–	Smooth muscle actin; a protein that is encoded by the *ACTA2* gene. It is a marker of smooth muscle differentiation. Similar function has smooth muscle myosin heavy chain marker (SMM-HC). Both proteins have diagnostic utility by immunohistochemistry.
SMARC4	–	SWI/SNF related, matrix associated, actin dependent regulator of chromatin, subfamily a, member 4; a gene that it mutated in small cell undifferentiated carcinoma, hypercalcemic type, and is considered to be a molecular signature of this malignancy.
STIC	–	Serous tubal intraepithelial carcinoma, the precursor of invasive high-grade serous carcinoma.
STIL	–	Serous tubal intraepithelial lesion; a term used by some pathologists for the same lesions as STIN.
STIN	–	Serous tubal intraepithelial neoplasia (low-grade) a p53 positive multilayered lesions which shows pseudo-stratification but only mild atypia and no loss of polarity

STK11	–	Serine threonine kinase, also known as liver kinase B1, LKB; gene encoding this protein is mutated in Peutz-Jeghers syndrome.
TDLU	–	Terminal duct lobular unit, the functional unit of the breast gland.
TP53	–	Tumor suppressor gene encoding p53
TSC2	–	Tuberous sclerosis 2 gene encoding the protein tuberin is inactivated in most perivascular epithelioid cell tumors.
UDH	–	Usual ductal hyperplasia
VUE	–	Villitis of unknown etiology
WT1	–	Wilms tumor suppressor gene 1
YWHAE-FAM22	–	A fusion gene found in high-grade endometrial stromal sarcomas, but not in low-grade ESS and endometrioid stromal nodules. *YWHAE* gene also known as 14-3-3ε, belongs to the family of 14-3-3 proteins—a gene encoding for a protein that belongs to the family of 14-3-3 proteins. It regulates signal transduction and has many cellular functions. By forming a fusion gene with *FAM22* it becomes oncogenic.

CHAPTER 1

Vulva, Vagina and Cervix

Q.1 A 3 cm well-circumscribed superficial submucosal, white tan and rubbery mass was removed from the vulva of a 35-year old woman (Figure 1.1). What is the most likely diagnosis?

A. Angiomyofibroblastoma
B. Deep angiomyxoma
C. Cellular angiofibroma
D. Superficial angiomyxoma
E. Fibroepithelial stromal polyp

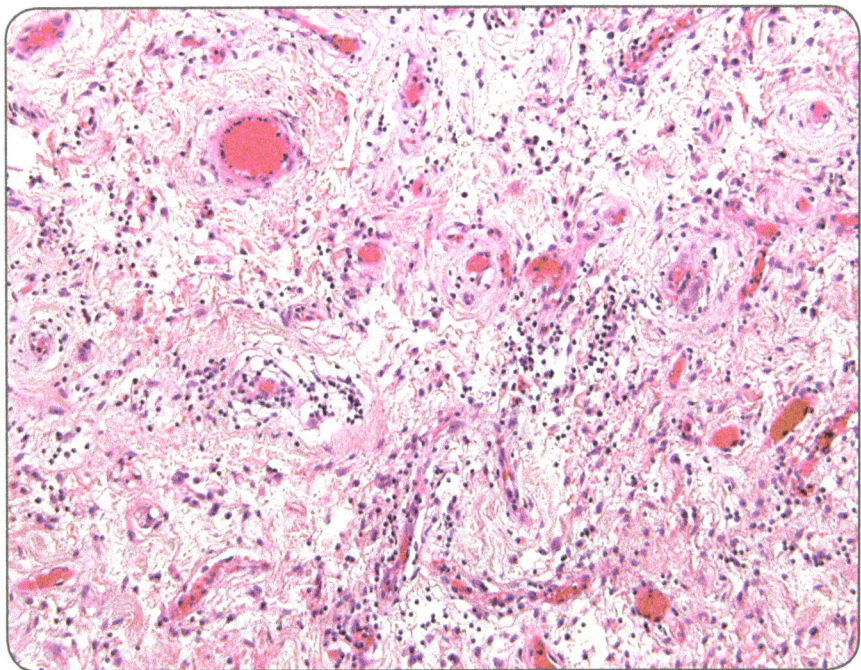

Figure 1.1

Answer: A. Angiomyofibroblastoma

Comment: All the tumors listed here occur in adult women of reproductive age. All of them are benign except deep angiomyxoma which has a tendency to recur locally in one-third of all cases.

Angiomyofibroblastoma is a benign well-circumscribed tumor of the vulva or vagina. Microscopically, it consists of alternating cellular areas centered around thin-walled blood vessels, and loosely structured ("myxoid") hypocellular areas.

Contd...

Contd...

Deep angiomyxoma is, as its name implies, a deeply seated and usually poorly demarcated perineal tumor. On gross examination, it is usually gelatinous, but older lesions and those previously biopsied or traumatized may be fibrotic. Microscopic features of this tumor may be deceptively innocuous because of the predominance of acellular myxoid matrix containing sparse spindle cells with bland nuclei. Scattered medium-sized or larger blood vessels are usually surrounded by condensed matrix and may have hyalinized walls.

Cellular angiofibroma is a benign vulvo-perineal tumor. It usually presents in the vulva as a small, circumscribed subcutaneous nodule. Microscopically, it appears uniformly homogenous and contains no myxoid areas. It consists of fibroblasts surrounded by collagen and scattered blood vessels ranging in size. Mitotic activity may be prominent but there is no nuclear atypia. Scattered mast cells may be conspicuous.

Superficial angiomyxoma usually presents as a gelatinous polypoid vulvar mass. Microscopically, it consists of hypocellular myxoid areas with thin-walled blood vessels. These neoplastic component may extend between the skin adnexa thus imparting the lesion a lobulated appearance.

Fibroepithelial stromal polyp may resemble warts or present as skin tag with a stalk. It may be found in the vulva, vagina or the cervix and is typically seen in pregnancy, or postmenopausal women taking hormones. They may be multiple, and tend to regress after pregnancy. The stromal core of these lesions is quite cellular, mitotically active. Underneath the surface squamous epithelium, the stroma may contain stellate or multinucleated large cells, which may be mistaken for malignancy.

Q.2 A 7 cm indistinctly demarcated perineal subepidermal myxoid mass was removed from the vulva of a 35-year-old woman (Figure 1.2). What is the most likely diagnosis?

    A. Angiomyofibroblastoma
    B. Deep angiomyxoma
    C. Cellular angiofibroma
    D. Superficial angiomyxoma
    E. Fibroepithelial stromal polyp

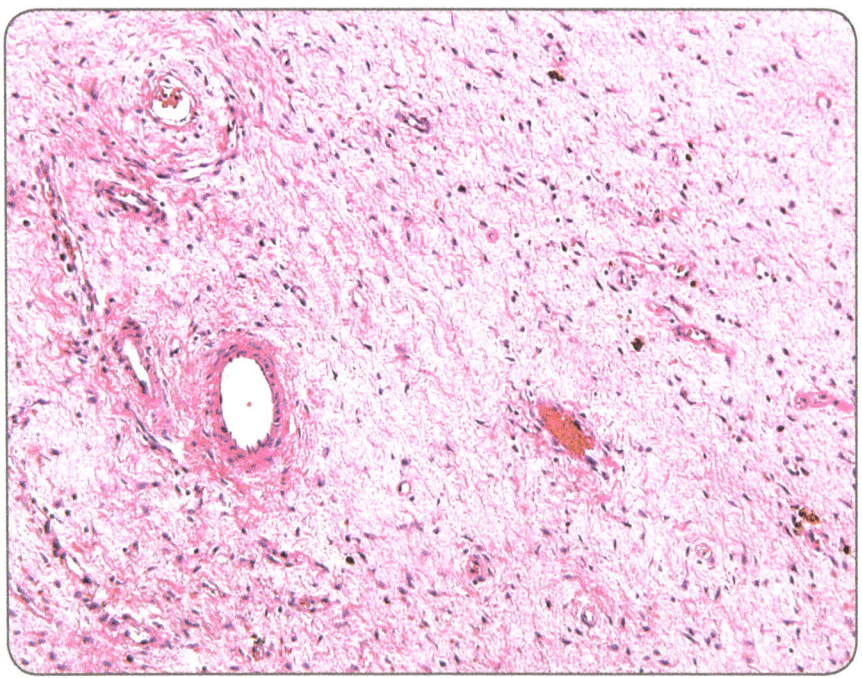

Figure 1.2

Answer: B. Deep angiomyxoma

Comment: **Deep angiomyxoma**, also known as **aggressive angiomyxoma** is a locally invasive tumor with indistinct borders. Incompletely resected tumors, which account for one-third of all deep angiomyxomas tend to recur, but even these tumors do not metastasize. See also the comment to question 1.

Q.3   Which of the following pathogens is the most likely cause of the wart like lesion shown in Figure 1.3?
   A. HPV-16 and HPV-18
   B. HPV-6 and HPV-11
   C. *Chlamydia trachomatis*
   D. *Treponema pallidum*
   E. Poxvirus

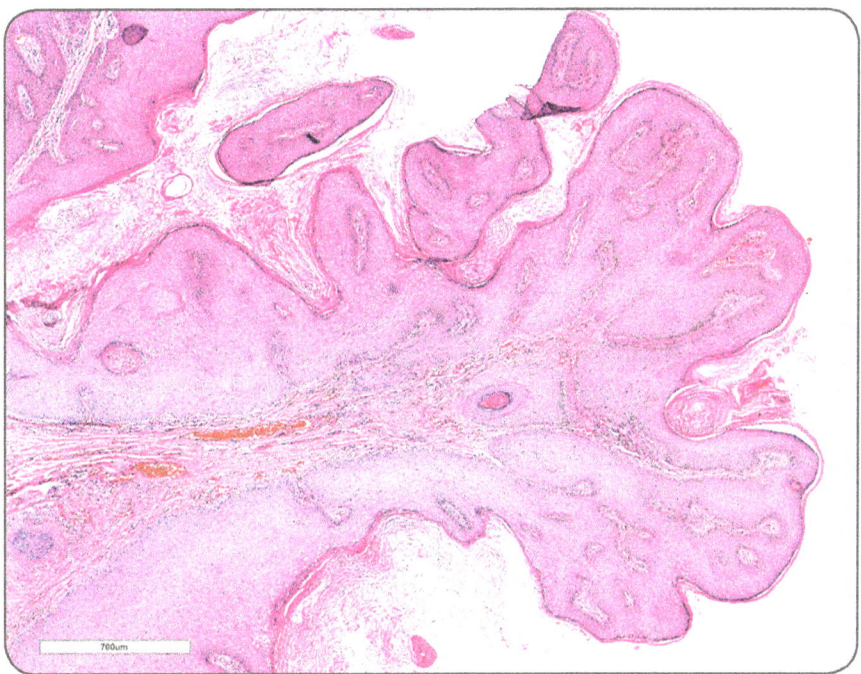

Figure 1.3

Answer: **B. HPV-6 and HPV-11**

Comment: **Genital wart** (*condyloma acuminatum*) shown in Figure 1.3 is caused by non-oncogenic human papilloma viruses **HPV types 6 and 11**. HPV types 16 and 18 are considered oncogenic, along with the type 31, 33, 45 HPV and several others, which are encountered less commonly. *Chlamydia trachomatis* causes acute genital infections and lymphogranuloma venereum, which is characterized by chronic inflammatory changes leading to skin erosion with lymph node enlargement, fibrosis and tissue destruction. *Treponema pallidum* is a causative agent of syphilis. **Condylomata lata** of syphilis present usually as plaques but also sometimes as flat warts. Poxvirus is a DNA virus causing **moluscum contagiosum**.

Q.4   Which of the following infections presents with small, smooth, centrally dimpled pearly-white vulvar papules containing microscopic intracytoplasmic eosinophilic bodies?
   A. Herpes simplex virus infection
   B. Varicella zoster virus infection
   C. Cytomegalovirus infection
   D. Molluscum contagiosum infection
   E. Non-oncogenic human papilloma virus infection

Answer: D. Molluscum contagiosum infection

Comment: **Molluscum contagiosum** infection presents clinically with pearly-white papules that show central umbillication. Microscopically, the infected cells contain eosinophilic intracytoplasmic bodies (Henderson-Paterson bodies).

Herpes virus infection presents with painful grouped vesicles. Microscopically, the infected cells show ballooning with formation of multinucleated keratinocytes and intranuclear ground glass inclusions.

Varicella zoster virus leads in adults to formation of grouped papules usually transforming into vesicles typical of shingles. Microscopic viral inclusions similar to those seen in herpetic lesions are seen in the necrotic tissue.

Cytomegalovirus infections present with nonspecific findings. Microscopically, the lesions contains enlarged infected cells with intranuclear and cytoplasmic inclusions containing numerous virions.

Non-oncogenic strains of HPV cause genital warts also know as condylomata acuminata.

Q.5 A 58-year-old woman was found to have white plaques on the labia minora bilaterally. A biopsy of the lesion is shown in Figure 1.4. What is the most likely diagnosis?
  A. Lichen planus
  B. Lichen sclerosus
  C. Lichen chronicus
  D. Drug reaction
  E. Morphea

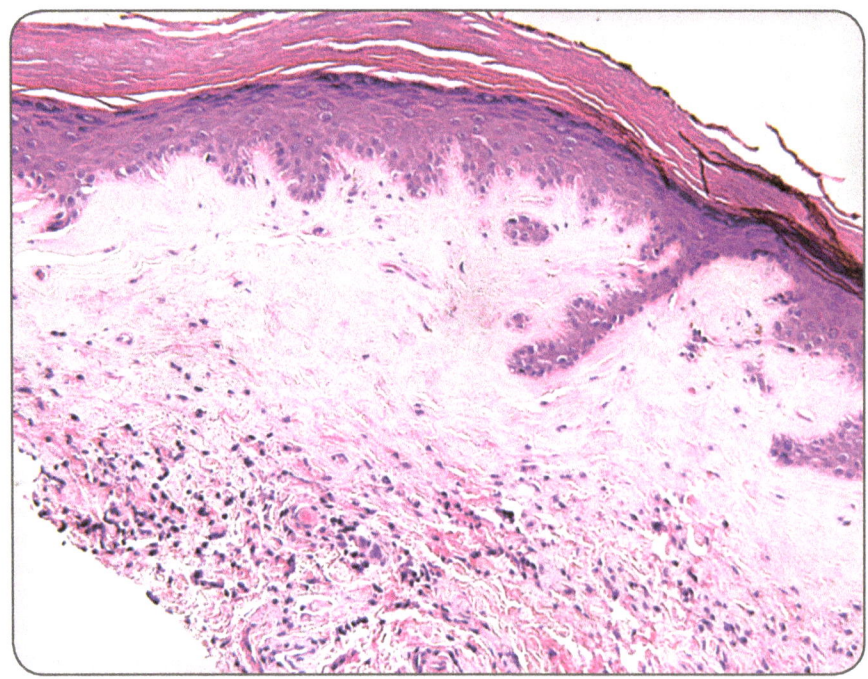

Figure 1.4

Answer: B. Lichen sclerosus

Comment: **Lichen sclerosus** (also known under its full Latin name as *lichen sclerosus et atrophicus*, LSA) is a fibrosing dermatitis of unknown etiology typically found on the vulva and anogenital skin of women. Initially, it presents with psoriasiform epithelial hyperplasia, hyperkeratosis, and a dermal lymphocytic infiltrate. With time the epithelium atrophies, the dermis become hyalinized and the lymphocytic infiltrates are pushed down and limited to the deep dermis, as shown in this Figure.

Contd...

Contd...

All other conditions listed in this question, except morphea, retain their inflammatory nature and do not undergo sclerosis. **Morphea**, a form of systemic sclerosis may involve the vulva. Histologically, the lesions show dense collagen bundles involving the deeper layers of the skin, which does not show the hyaline changes as in LSA.

Q.6 Which one of the following is a direct precursor of invasive vulvar squamous cell carcinoma?
   A. Lichen simplex chronicus
   B. Low grade vulvar intraepithelial neoplasia I (VIN I)
   C. Differentiated/simplex vulvar intraepithelial neoplasia
   D. Condyloma acuminatum
   E. Molluscum contagiosum

Answer: C. Differentiated/simplex vulvar intraepithelial neoplasia

Comment: **Vulvar intraepithelial neoplasia** (VIN 3) is divided into two histologic types: **classic** and **differentiated** (simplex). The latter is considered a high grade lesion, and has a potential of progressing into **squamous cell carcinoma**, despite its unremarkable architectural distortion and well-developed intracellular bridges. Nevertheless, cytological features, such as significant nuclear atypia and prominent nucleoli are more suggestive of its neoplastic nature. More differentiating features of classic and differentiated VIN are listed in Table 1.1.

Classic VIN is graded on the similar basis as cervical intraepithelial neoplasia (CIN), with the grade I involving dysplasia in the lower third of the epithelial thickness, and grade II and III dysplasia in two-thirds or full thickness of the epithelium.

Lichen simplex chronicus is characterized by chronic inflammation and collagenous bands ("vertical steaks") under the epidermis. It is not a premalignant lesion.

Condyloma acuminatum is usually papillary although it may occur in a flat form as well. It is caused by low-risk HPV types 6 and 11, and it is not considered to be preneoplastic.

Moluscum contagiosum is an infectious disease caused by a poxvirus and is not associated with an increased risk for cancer.

Table 1.1: Features of classic versus differentiated vulvar intraepithelial neoplasia (VIN)

	Classic VIN	*Differentiated VIN*
Prevalence	Common	Less common
Age	Younger women (30–50 years)	Postmenopausal (60+ years)
Distribution	Multifocal	Unifocal
Risk factors	HPV infection and HPV infection related risk factors	Chronic skin conditions (squamous hyperplasia or lichen sclerosus)
Type of squamous carcinoma	Warty, basaloid	Keratinizing
Morphology	Decreased maturation (undifferentiated, basophilic)	Premature maturation (deep keratinization, eosinophilic)
Immunoprofile	Diffuse p16+	p16- or focal+, p53+ (>80% cases)

Q.7 A 40-year-old woman complained of vulvar pruritus. Several white plaques were noted on the inner side of labia majora and were biopsied (Figure 1.5). What is the most likely diagnosis?
   A. Lichen simplex chronicus
   B. Low grade vulvar intraepithelial neoplasia I (VIN I)
   C. Differentiated/simplex vulvar intraepithelial neoplasia
   D. Classic vulvar intraepithelial neoplasia (VIN 3)
   E. Moluscum contagiosum

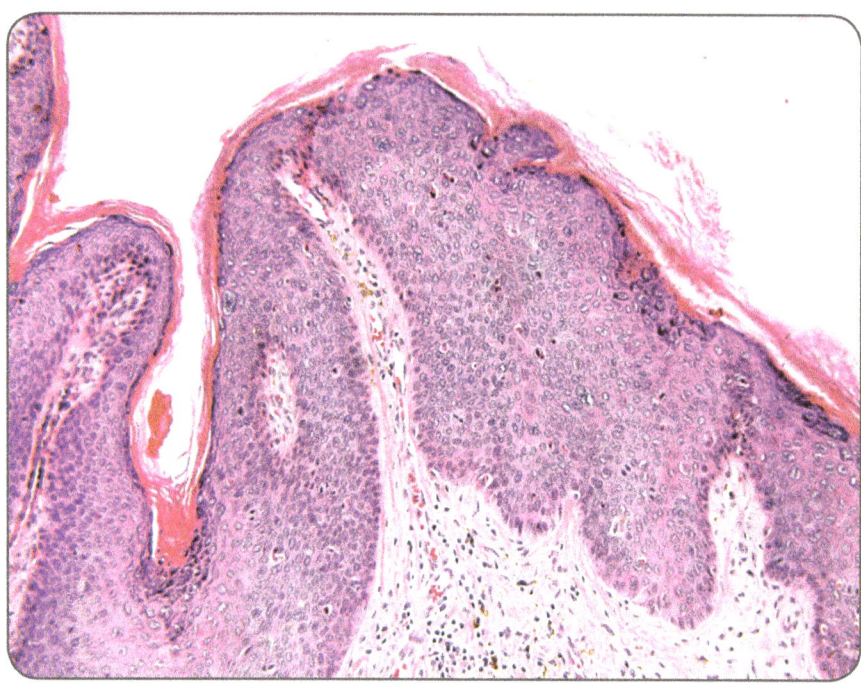

Figure 1.5

Answer: D. Classic vulvar intraepithelial neoplasia (VIN 3)

Comment: The biopsy shows typical microscopic features of classical VIN 3. The epithelium is thickened with surface keratosis and parakeratosis but otherwise lacking mostly any maturation. The entire lesion appears bluish due to a high nuclear to cytoplasmic ratio of neoplastic cells, which also show marked hyperchromasia and nuclear crowding.

Q.8 A 65-year-old woman presented with an itchy, erythematous plaque on her left labium persisting for more than one year. The lesion was excised. Histological examination revealed squamous epithelium containing isolated neoplastic cells with abundant pale cytoplasm and prominent nucleoli, involving basal and parabasal layers of epithelium. The cytoplasm of neoplastic cells stained with PAS and immunohistochemically with the antibody to cytokeratin CK7. What is the most likely diagnosis?

   A. Vulvar melanoma
   B. Vulvar intraepithelial neoplasia (VIN)
   C. Lichen sclerosus et atrophicus
   D. Condyloma latum
   E. Extramammary Paget disease

Answer: E. Extramammary Paget disease

Comment: This biopsy shows the typical microscopic features of **extramammary Paget disease (EMPD)**. It is an uncommon form of malignancy that most often involves the vulva. In 25% cases it is associated with an underlying malignancy of the gastrointestinal or urogenital tract. These lesions, as well those that show extensive involvement of vulvar epithelium have poor prognosis.

Melanoma is the most important malignancy that must be distinguished from EMPD. It is a much more lethal and more aggressive neoplasm. Its cells do not contain mucin, therefore, the lesion does not stain with the periodic Schiff (PAS) reaction. Melanoma does not react with antibodies to cytokeratin 7, but is positive for melanoma markers (HMB45 and MART1).

Condylomata lata (note that this is the correct Latin plural of condyloma latum, in singular!) are caused by *Treponema pallidum* and the patient typically has other signs of syphilis.

Contd...

Contd...

Lichen sclerosus et atrophicus is characterized by thinning of the epithelium with a damaged basal layer, and hyalinization of the dermal connective tissue rimmed at the base by a chronic inflammatory infiltrate.

Vulvar intraepithelial neoplasia (VIN) in its classical or differentiated form has a different architectural and cytological appearance (*see* Figure 1.5).

Q.9 All the following statements about vulvar carcinoma are true, *except*:
   A. Leukoplakia is a diagnostic feature of vulvar carcinoma
   B. Vulvar carcinoma may be HPV related or non-HPV related
   C. HPV related vulvar carcinoma originates from dysplastic precursor lesion called classical VIN
   D. Non-HPV related carcinoma usually arises from dysplastic precursor called differentiated VIN
   E. HPV related carcinomas occur in younger women than non-HPV related carcinoma

Answer: A. Leukoplakia is a specific sign of vulvar carcinoma

Comment: **Leukoplakia** is a nonspecific finding and may be found in several dysplastic, neoplastic and inflammatory conditions. Biopsy is often required to distinguish carcinoma from other causes. HPV related carcinomas arise due to infection with high-risk HPV types 16 and 18, causing dysplastic precursor lesions (VIN), which includes koilocytic change, nuclear atypia, disordered maturation and increased mitotic activity. It usually affects premenopausal women with risk factors such as young age of first sexual intercourse, frequent change of partners, etc. Non-HPV related carcinoma occurs predominantly in postmenopausal women. It arises from differentiated VIN, and in a minority of cases it may be even related to lichen sclerosus.

Q.10 A 60-year-old woman presented with the pain and swelling in the genital region. Physical examination revealed a painful, fluctuating mass on her left labia, measuring 4.5 cm. The lesion was excised and sent for histopathological examination. Representative section is shown on the Figure 1.6. What is the most likely diagnosis?
   A. Vulvar intraepithelial neoplasia 3 (VIN 3)
   B. Lichen sclerosus
   C. Squamous cell carcinoma
   D. Herpes simplex infection
   E. Bartholin gland cyst

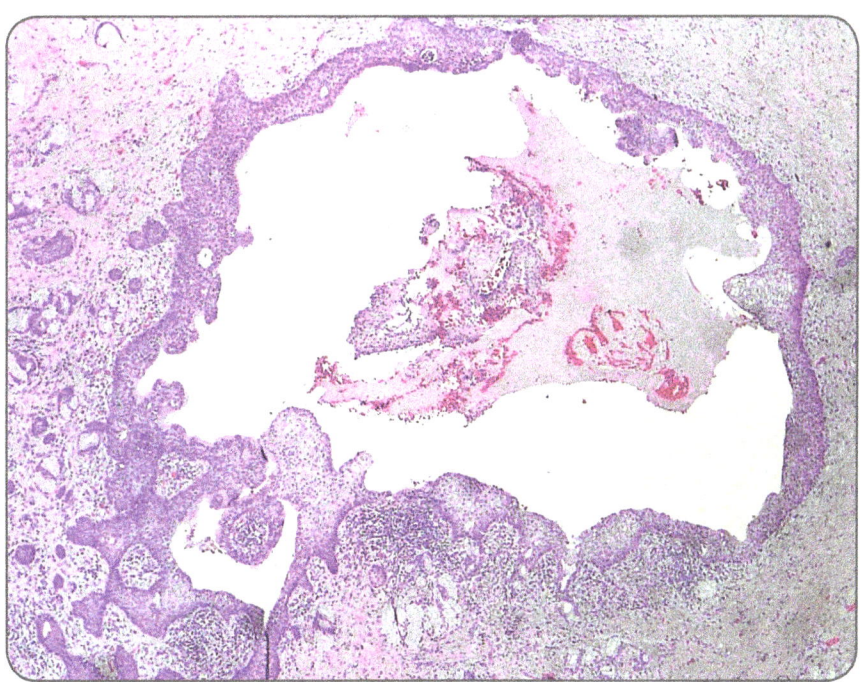

Figure 1.6

Answer: E. Bartholin gland cyst

Comment: **Bartholin cysts** occur after Bartholin duct obstruction. The epithelium lining the cyst may be squamous (as is in this case), transitional, or low cuboidal mucinous. The inflammatory response within the adjacent tissue may be minimal or nonexistent. Bartholin cysts may recur if not completely removed. In postmenopausal women, some recurrent cysts or palpable masses remaining after cyst drainage may harbor carcinoma and such tumor need to be widely excised.

Q.11 A 7-year-old girl has been referred to her physician for "blood on her underwear". The physical examination revealed a well-circumscribed polypoid mass on the posterior wall of her vagina, measuring 1 cm. The lesion was removed and histological examination showed papillary fronds lined by cuboidal cells with uniform, bland nuclei and no mitotic activity. Stromal cores were composed of fibrovascular tissue showing focal edema. What is the most likely diagnosis?

A. Fibroepithelial-stromal polyp
B. Condyloma acuminatum
C. Müllerian papilloma
D. Embryonal rhabdomyosarcoma
E. Clear cell carcinoma

Answer: C. Müllerian papilloma

Comment: **Müllerian papilloma** is a rare polypoid benign vaginal tumor of infants and children. Microscopically, it is composed of a fibrovascular core lined on its surface by bland cuboidal epithelium, which is thought to be of Müllerian origin.

Fibroepithelial-stromal polyp is composed of fibrovascular stroma containing stellate and multinucleated cells. On its surface, it is tightly covered by squamous epithelium that may show variable degrees hyperplasia, but no atypia. Fibroepithelial-stromal polyps do not occur in children; they are most often found in women during pregnancy or those on hormone replacement therapy.

Condyloma acuminatum is lined by squamous epithelium and is unlikely in children, unless sexual abuse and HPV infection is suspected.

Embryonal rhabdomyosarcoma is composed of myxoid, lose or dense stroma and cellular regions of small, undifferentiated, primitive cells with interspersed rhabdo-myoblasts. A so called cambium layer of rhabdomyoblasts can be seen in the subepithelial portion of the tumor.

Clear cell carcinoma shows tubular, papillary or solid architecture with marked nuclear atypia and frequent mitotic figures.

Q.12 Which of the following vaginal lesions is characterized by a high mitotic count?

A. Postoperative spindle cell nodule
B. Vaginal vault granulation tissue
C. Endometriosis
D. Fallopian tube prolapse
E. Vaginal adenosis

Answer: A. Postoperative spindle cell nodule

Comment: All the lesions listed in this question may present as visible or palpable masses and are sometimes listed under the heading of **pseudoneoplastic lesions of the vagina.**

Postoperative spindle cell nodule is characterized by spindle cells arranged in a fascicular pattern, with minimal cytologic atypia, but high mitotic count (up to 25/10 HPFs). Delicate network of small blood vessels is present, as well as limited infiltration into adjacent tissue.

Granulation tissue presents as elsewhere in the body, with prominent small blood vessels, edema, and marked chronic inflammation.

Contd...

Contd...

> **Endometriosis** presents with endometrial-type glands in endometrial stroma, and recent hemorrhage or hemosiderin in the stroma and macrophages.
> **Fallopian tube prolapse** most commonly occurs following a vaginal hysterectomy, but it can also occur after abdominal hysterectomy or colpotomy.
> **Vaginal adenosis** presents with glands lined by endocervical or tubal or endometrioid-type epithelium. Such epithelium may focally replace surface squamous epithelium of the vagina or form tubular glands in the stroma.

Q.13 All the following statements about the high-grade vaginal intraepithelial neoplasia (HGVAIN) are correct, *except:*
   A. Usually affects postmenopausal women
   B. Vaginal atrophy is a precursor lesion of HGVAIN
   C. Transitional cell metaplasia is mimicker of HGVAIN
   D. Nuclear pleomorphism and hyperchromasia involve the lower two-thirds or full thickness of the epithelium
   E. Immunohistochemically p16 and Ki-67 expression is strongly positive

Answer: B. Vaginal atrophy is a precursor lesion of HGVAIN

Comment: **Vaginal atrophy** is not a precursor lesion of HGVAIN. The epithelium in vaginal atrophy is usually thinner than in HGVAIN. Cells in vaginal atrophy show nuclear hyperchromasia and increased nuclear to cytoplasmic ratio, but nuclei do not show significant pleomorphism and mitotic figures are scarce.

Q.14 A 29-year-old pregnant woman with a biopsy proven history of cervical low grade squamous intraepithelial lesion had a cervical biopsy. The biopsy revealed nests and sheets of large, polygonal, eosinophilic cells in the stroma, with bland nuclei and no mitotic figures. Immunohistochemical staining for cytokeratin gave negative results. What is the most likely diagnosis?
   A. Invasive squamous cell carcinoma
   B. Immature squamous cell hyperplasia
   C. Arias-Stella reaction
   D. Decidual reaction
   E. Microglandular hyperplasia

Answer: D. Decidual reaction

Comment: **Decidual reaction** of pregnancy may involve the cervix, fallopian tubes, foci of endometriosis and peritoneum. This decidual reaction involving the cervical stroma may be mistaken for invasive squamous cell carcinoma. However, decidualized cells lack nuclear atypia and show no mitotic activity. Negative immunoreactivity for cytokeratin should help in distinguishing decidual reaction from squamous cell carcinoma.
   Arias-Stella reaction is a pregnancy-related reaction producing nuclear atypia of cells within endometrial glands. It may be associated with gestation, gestational trophoblastic disease, treatment with gonadotropins or progestins. Typically, it involves endometrial glands but it may be seen in the endocervix and even in foci of cervicovaginal adenosis.
   Immature squamous metaplasia shows an increased nuclear/cytoplasmic ratio; a lack of maturation combined with hyperchromasia could lead to an erroneous diagnosis of cervical dysplasia. However, the nuclei in immature squamous metaplasia are uniform with smooth nuclear contours. Mitotic figures are rarely present and if present appear normal. Ki-67 should stain no more than 15% of the parabasal or surface cells in case of squamous metaplasia.
   Microglandular hyperplasia is typically associated with pregnancy or oral contraceptives. It consists of closely packed glands of variable size and shape, with little intervening stroma. In contrast to adenocarcinoma, there is no nuclear hyperchromasia or atypia.

Q.15 What is the percentage of high-grade squamous epithelial lesions (HSIL) that will eventually progress to invasive carcinoma?

    A. 100%
    B. 80%
    C. 50%
    D. 20%
    E. 10%

Answer: E. 10%

Comment: About 10% of **high-grade squamous epithelial lesions (HSIL)** will eventually progress to invasive carcinoma within 10 years. Similarly, 10% of low-grade squamous intraepithelial lesions (LSIL) will progress to HSIL. About 60% of LSIL regress and 30% persist, in contrast to HSIL where 30% regress and 60% persist. Hence, the difference in therapeutic approach: LSIL is managed conservatively and deserves clinical follow-up, while HSIL is treated by surgical excision.

Q.16 What is the best diagnosis for the cervical lesion shown in Figure 1.7?

    A. Low-grade squamous intraepithelial lesion, (CIN 1)
    B. High-grade squamous intraepithelial lesion, (CIN 2)
    C. High-grade squamous intraepithelial lesion, (CIN 3)
    D. Squamous metaplasia
    E. Invasive squamous cell carcinoma

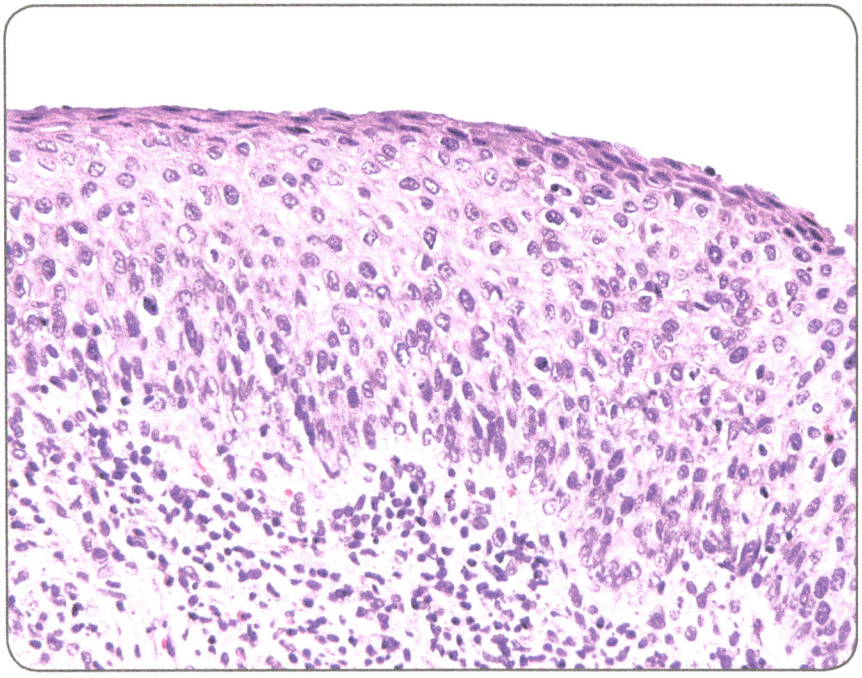

Figure 1.7

Answer: C. **High-grade squamous intraepithelial lesion, (CIN 3)**

Comment: **High-grade squamous intraepithelial lesion, (CIN 3)** shows thickening of the cervical epithelium which contains atypical hyperchromatic cells in all its layers, including the surface parakeratotic layer.

Q.17 Cervical intraepithelial neoplasia III (CIN 3) is characterized by all the following, *except*:

A. Loss of maturation through the full thickness of the epithelium
B. Immature cells with high nuclear/cytoplasmic ratio, irregular nuclear membrane contour, coarse chromatin, and inconspicuous nucleoli
C. Frequent mitoses, including atypical forms
D. Strong and diffuse positive nuclear and cytoplasmic p16 in at least two-thirds of the epithelial thickness
E. Paradoxical keratinization

Answer: E. Paradoxical keratinization

Comment: **Paradoxical keratinization** is a phenomenon associated with superficially invasive squamous cell carcinoma. Namely, the immature neoplastic cells disrupting the basal membrane and invading the stroma, acquire more abundant, eosinophilic cytoplasm, prominent nucleoli, and well-defined cell borders. This phenomenon may be helpful in distinguishing HSIL and invasive squamous cell carcinoma in the tissue altered by artifacts or in poorly oriented tissue.

Q.18 Which of the following lesion mimicking high-grade squamous intraepithelial lesion (HSIL) is more often found in postmenopausal women rather than in women of reproductive age?

A. Transitional metaplasia
B. Reactive atypia
C. Immature squamous metaplasia
D. Low-grade squamous intraepithelial lesion
E. Radiation changes

Answer: A. Transitional metaplasia

Comment: **Transitional metaplasia** occurs predominantly in postmenopausal women. It can involve the transformation zone, the exocervix, as well as the vagina. It is typically more than 10 cell layers thick and thus may resemble **high-grade squamous intraepithelial lesion (HSIL).** Furthermore there is no maturation, and the nuclei are oval and have irregular contours. However, in contrast to HSIL, the cells in the superficial layers are oriented horizontally, the nuclei are elongated, and mitoses are rare.
Immature squamous metaplasia, LSIL and radiation changes may occur in patients of any age and are not more common in postmenopausal than in menopausal women.

Q.19 All the following are found in high-grade squamous intraepithelial neoplasia but not in low-grade squamous intraepithelial neoplasia, *except*:

A. Atypical mitoses and mitoses in the upper two-thirds of the epithelium
B. Extension of basaloid cells above the lower third of epithelium
C. Disorderly arrangement of cells in the lower third of epithelium
D. Positive p16 immunohistochemical staining through the entire thickness of epithelium
E. Koilocytosis of the superficial and intermediate layer cells

Answer: C. Koilocytosis of the superficial and intermediate layer cells

Comment: **Koilocytosis** is a sign of **active HPV infection**, and may appear in any form or degree of dysplasia. However, koilocytosis is more common in LSIL than in HSIL, because the increased dysplasia, not the infection, becomes the major pathogenetic mechanism in HSIL. Extension of basaloid cells into the upper layers and disorderly arrangement of cells in the lower third layer are characteristic features of HSIL. Immunohistochemical staining for p16 has been the major surrogate for HPV detection; it shows diffuse positivity of the entire epithelial layer in HSIL.

Q.20 Which of the following changes is related to reduced serum levels of estrogen in postmenopausal women?

- A. Low-grade squamous intraepithelial lesion, (CIN 1)
- B. High-grade squamous intraepithelial lesion, (CIN 2)
- C. High-grade squamous intraepithelial lesion, (CIN 3)
- D. Reactive atypia
- E. Atrophy of cervical epithelium

Answer: E. Atrophy of cervical epithelium

Comment: **Atrophy of cervical epithelium** is a consequence of low serum levels of estrogen in postmenopausal women. Atrophic epithelium lacks significant nuclear pleomorphism, and shows no significant mitotic activity. However, in some cases of atrophy cells may show enlarged nuclei with pleomorphism which make it hard to distinguish from HSIL. Ki-67 and p16 stains will be helpful in such cases. The cells in the atrophic epithelium are p16 negative and Ki-67 expression is either negative or restricted to the basal and parabasal layers.

Reactive atypia is usually associated with a stromal inflammatory infiltrate.

Squamous intraepithelial lesions do not develop faster in women with low estrogen levels than in those with normal estrogen levels or hyperestrinemia.

Q.21 Which anatomic part of the cervix is considered to be most susceptible to HPV infection?

- A. Endocervix
- B. Exocervix
- C. Transformation zone
- D. Internal cervical orifice
- E. External cervical orifice

Answer: C. Transformation zone

Comment: HPV has the highest affinity for the cells of **transformation zone of the cervix,** although, infection may occur on any damaged cervical site.

Q.22 HPV gene products bind and interact with many targets within the host human cells, but two of the targets are particularly important, since they are tumor suppressor genes and have regulatory function in cell cycle, proliferation and programmed cell death. Which proteins are they?

- A. HER2 and estrogen receptor
- B. *BRCA1* and *BRCA2*
- C. p53 and pRb
- D. WT1 and PTEN
- E. None of the above

Answer: C. p53 and pRb

Comment: The role of **p53 and pRb** (retinoblastoma protein) in cervical carcinoma pathogenesis has been well-documented. The binding of HPV E6 to human p53 results in the blocking of apoptosis, and the binding of E7 to the retinoblastoma tumor suppression protein pRb abolishes cell-cycle arrest leading to uncontrolled cellular proliferation.

Q.23 Which of the following is the best term for multiple small mucinous cysts of the endocervix that result from blockage of the endocervical glands by overlying squamous metaplastic epithelium?

A. Gartner duct cysts
B. Bartholin cysts
C. Chocolate cysts
D. Follicular cysts
E. Nabothian cysts

Answer: E. Nabothian cysts

Comment: **Nabothian cysts** are the most common type of cyst of the cervix. They develop within the transformation zone due to **squamous metaplasia**, covering over and obstructing **endocervical glands**.
Gartner duct cysts, also termed mesonephric cysts, are most often located along the anterolateral wall of the vagina, following the route of the mesonephric duct.
Bartholin cysts occur due to obstruction of duct exiting Bartholin gland of the vulva, causing accumulation of gland fluid. Follicular cysts are benign cysts of the ovary.
Chocolate cysts is a colloquial term for hemorrhagic cystic foci of endometriosis of the ovary. The brownish-red color of the material inside these cysts is usually derived from hemosiderin and hemolyzed red blood cells.

Q.24 A 35-year-old woman with a history of two previous pregnancies and two abortions, 5-year-long use of oral contraceptives, and treatment for vaginosis, was referred to her gynecologist for intermittent bleeding after sexual intercourse. On colposcopy, a flat reddish lesion is found on her cervix, and sampled for histology. The diagnosis of microglandular hyperplasia was established. Which one of the following clinical data is the most supportive of the diagnosis?

A. Previous pregnancy
B. Previous abortion
C. Use of oral contraceptives
D. Vaginosis
E. Endocervical polyp

Answer: C. Use of oral contraceptives

Comment: **Microglandular endocervical hyperplasia** is usually induced by oral contraceptives. Most often it is an incidental finding on a cervical biopsy, cone biopsy or a hysterectomy specimens. Tightly packed "back to back" benign endocervical glands, age of the patient, and history of contraceptive usage are all features of these lesions. If clinically apparent, it most often resembles **a cervical polyp**. These glandular lesions do not show microscopically any atypia, or mitotic activity. Inflammatory infiltrates are usually present but are not diagnostic.

Q.25 A 31-year-old woman is referred to her gynecologist for painful and prolonged menstrual cycles and intermittent postcoital bleeding. The colposcopy showed a red nodule on her cervix, which was biopsied (Figure 1.8). What is the most likely diagnosis?

A. Endocervical adenocarcinoma in situ
B. Microglandular hyperplasia
C. Cervical endometriosis
D. Lobular glandular hyperplasia
E. High-grade serous uterine carcinoma

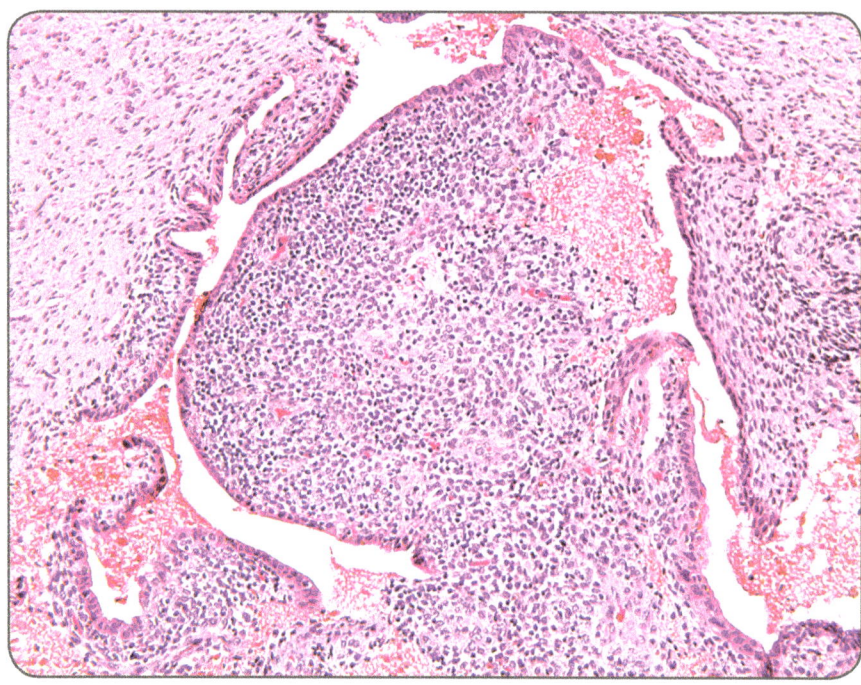

Figure 1.8

Answer: **C. Cervical endometriosis**

Comment: **Endometriosis** represents ectopic **endometrial glands and stroma.** Endometriosis of the cervix may occur on the vaginal portion or in the endocervical canal. Histologically, the glands and stroma resemble proliferative endometrium, but occasionally they may be secretory. The stroma contains extravasated blood and deposits of hemosiderin.

Decidua may be seen in pregnancy or following progestin therapy. Decidual cells have eosinophilic cytoplasm and bland nuclei.

Endocervical adenocarcinoma in situ usually shows nuclear atypia and although it may occur in several microscopic forms, the cells of the most common endocervical type usually contain some mucin and react strongly with the antibody to p16.

Microglandular and lobular glandular hyperplasia show tightly packed small or variably sized glands, respectively. The nuclei or these glands have a bland appearance.

High-grade serous uterine carcinoma shows significant atypia, hyperchromatic nuclei, prominent myometrial invasion, frequent mitotic activity, necrosis, marked desmoplastic response.

Q.26 What is the most common benign cervical lesion discovered in adult women during routine vaginal gynecologic examination?

    A. Endocervical polyp
    B. Granulation tissue
    C. Mesodermal stromal polyp
    D. Placental site nodule
    E. Cervical leiomyoma

Answer: **A. Endocervical polyp**

Comment: **Endocervical polyps** represent the most common mass lesion in the cervix. They usually occur in women in age fourth to six decade.

Granulation tissue may have polypoid features. Microscopically, granulation tissue is characterized by proliferation of newly-formed blood vessels and chronic inflammation.

Contd...

Contd...

Mesodermal stromal polyp is composed of an edematous stroma covered by a benign stratified squamous epithelium. Stromal cells are mainly the fibroblast, which sometimes may show significant atypia.

Placental site trophoblastic nodules are composed of intermediate trophoblast with prominent hyalinization, and some chronic inflammation. The intermediate trophoblast cells are frequently degenerated and show extensive cytoplasmic vacuolization but lack significant nuclear atypia, mitotic activity. Immunohistochemically, they are positive for human placental lactogen, and the staining for Ki-67 shows low proliferative activity.

Cervical leiomyomas are much less common than their uterine counterparts. These tumors are composed of spindle shaped cells with all the usual features of smooth muscle cells with no nuclear atypia.

Q.27 A 65-year-old paid a visit to the gynecologist complaining of spotty vaginal bleeding. Colposcopy revealed a polypoid lesion (Figure 1.9). What is the most likely diagnosis?

A. Cervical hemangioma
B. Nabothian cyst
C. Adenocarcinoma
D. Endocervical polyp
E. Endometriosis

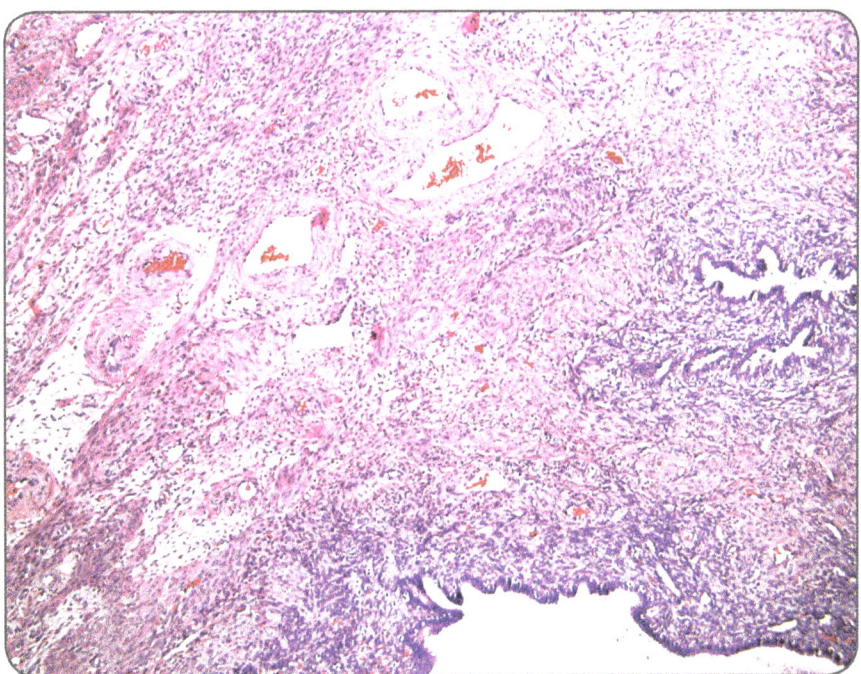

Figure 1.9

Answer: D. Endocervical polyp

Comment: Endocervical polyps contain endocervical glands surrounded by moderately cellular stroma, which in part may by collagenized containing **thick-walled blood vessels.**

Nabothian cyst occurs due to blockade of the endocervical glands by the metaplastic squamous cell epithelium.

Adenocarcinoma of the cervix shows the usual signs of malignancy, such as nuclear atypia, hyperchromasia, architectural distortion of glands, which are typically surrounded by a desmoplastic reaction.

Cervical hemangioma has the usual features of vascular tumors in other sites, and is usually classified as capillary or cavernous.

Endometriosis is microscopically composed of cycling or atrophic endometrial glands and endometrial type stroma, with foci of hemorrhage and hemosiderin deposition.

Q.28 Which of the following is the most common subtype of cervical adenocarcinoma in situ (AIS)?

A. Endocervical type
B. Intestinal type
C. Endometrioid type
D. Adenosquamous type
E. Clear cell type

Answer: A. Endocervical type

Comment: **Cervical adenocarcinoma in situ (AIS)** is also known as high-grade cervical glandular intraepithelial neoplasia (HG-CGIN). The most common microscopic form of AIS is the **endocervical type,** i.e. the one that resembles normal endocervical glands the most. It may be admixed to other types which are classified as follows: **endometrioid, intestinal, adenosquamous, tubal or clear cell types.** The last two types are very rare. These microscopic variants do not have any clinical or biological significance and are important only for histopathologic diagnosis purposes.

Q.29 A cervical adenocarcinoma was diagnosed upon histologic examination of the hysterectomy specimen. The tumor had a complex architecture and was focally cribriform and papillary. The columnar cells lining the neoplastic glands had pseudostratified nuclei and variable amounts of mucus rich cytoplasm. Immunohistochemically, the cells were p16 and CEA positive. This tumor is best considered to be which subtype of cervical adenocarcinoma?

A. Usual endocervical
B. Intestinal
C. Endometrioid
D. Adenosquamous
E. Clear cell

Answer: A. Usual endocervical

Comment: This tumor is composed of cells that resemble normal endocervical glands infected with HPV, and are thus CEA and p16 positive. It is thus classified as **usual endocervical** type adenocarcinoma.

Q.30 A cervical adenocarcinoma was diagnosed. It contained numerous goblet cells which were immunohistochemically positive for MUC2. This tumor is best considered to be which subtype of endocervical adenocarcinoma?

A. Endocervical
B. Intestinal
C. Endometrioid
D. Adenosquamous
E. Clear cell

Answer: B. Intestinal

Comment: Goblet cells that are MUC2 positive are a hallmark of **intestinal endocervical adenocarcinoma.**

Vulva, Vagina and Cervix

Q.31 Which immunohistochemical stain if positive is most useful for confirming the diagnosis of cervical adenocarcinoma in situ?

A. p16
B. p53
C. p63
D. bcl-2
E. Vimentin

Answer: **A. p16**

Comment: Vast majority of **cervical adenocarcinomas in situ (AIS)** are caused by HPV and thus **p16** positive, whereas other immunostains listed here are mostly negative or show only focal reactivity with some neoplastic cells. Another useful immunohistochemical stain is MIB-1 (Ki-67) which usually shows in AIS a proliferative index exceeding 30%.

Q.32 All the following statements about invasive cervical squamous cell carcinoma are true, *except*:

A. Tumor is called microinvasive and has better prognosis if tumor diameter is <7 mm and depth of invasion <3 mm
B. Desmoplastic reaction is helpful when evaluating invasion of the tumor
C. Atypical mitotic figures are numerous and readily identifiable
D. Tumor grading is based on the presence or absence of prominent nucleoli
E. Tumors are cytokeratin and p63 positive

Answer: **D. Tumor grading is based on the presence or absence of prominent nucleoli**

Comment: To grade cervical squamous cell carcinoma one must assess the extent of **keratinization** within the tumor. Tumors forming keratin pearls are considered well-differentiated, while tumors lacking keratin formation are considered high-grade. Desmoplastic reaction is one of the most helpful features in recognizing tumor invasion, and combined with paradoxical keratinization may prove very helpful in distinguishing extensive squamous cell metaplasia or carcinoma in situ from invasive squamous cell carcinoma.

Q.33 Which of the following forms of cervical adenocarcinoma has a generally poor prognosis?

A. Adenocarcinoma, usual type
B. Villoglandular adenocarcinoma
C. Endometrioid adenocarcinoma
D. Adenocarcinoma, intestinal type
E. Adenocarcinoma, gastric type

Answer: **E. Adenocarcinoma, gastric type**

Comment: **Adenocarcinomas of the gastric type** have a generally poor prognosis, in part due to the advanced stage at diagnosis. Overall villoglandular carcinomas have the best prognosis, whereas all others have approximately similar clinical features depending on the grade, stage and lymph node involvement.

Q.34 What is the most likely diagnosis of this endocervical carcinoma removed from a 30-year-old woman (Figure 1.10)?

A. Adenocarcinoma, usual type
B. Villoglandular adenocarcinoma
C. Endometrioid adenocarcinoma
D. Adenocarcinoma, intestinal type
E. Adenocarcinoma, gastric type

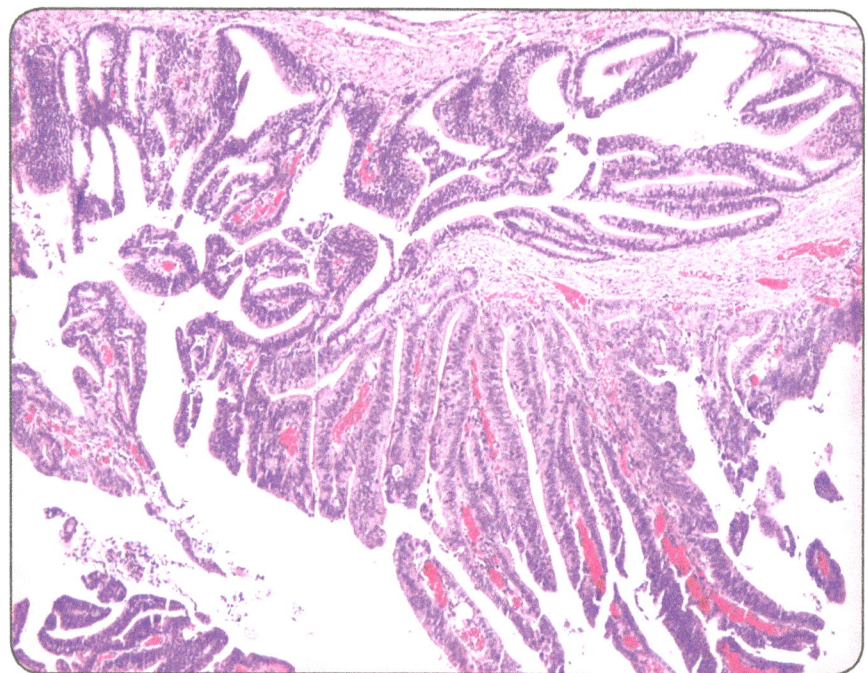

Figure 1.10

Answer: B. Villoglandular adenocarcinoma

Comment: This **villoglandular carcinoma** forms papillae and invaginates into gland-like structures lined by epithelium showing only mild atypia. This epithelium has endometrial features, albeit in some tumors it may resemble endocervical epithelium and even have enteric features. Villoglandular carcinoma is typically found in young women. It is only superficially invasive and it has a good prognosis.

Q.35 An invasive carcinoma was noted in the cervix invading into the lateral sides of the muscle layer. The tumor was GATA3 positive. What is the most likely diagnosis for this tumor shown in Figure 1.11?

A. Adenocarcinoma, usual type
B. Villoglandular adenocarcinoma

C. Endometrioid adenocarcinoma
D. Adenocarcinoma, intestinal type
E. Mesonephric adenocarcinoma

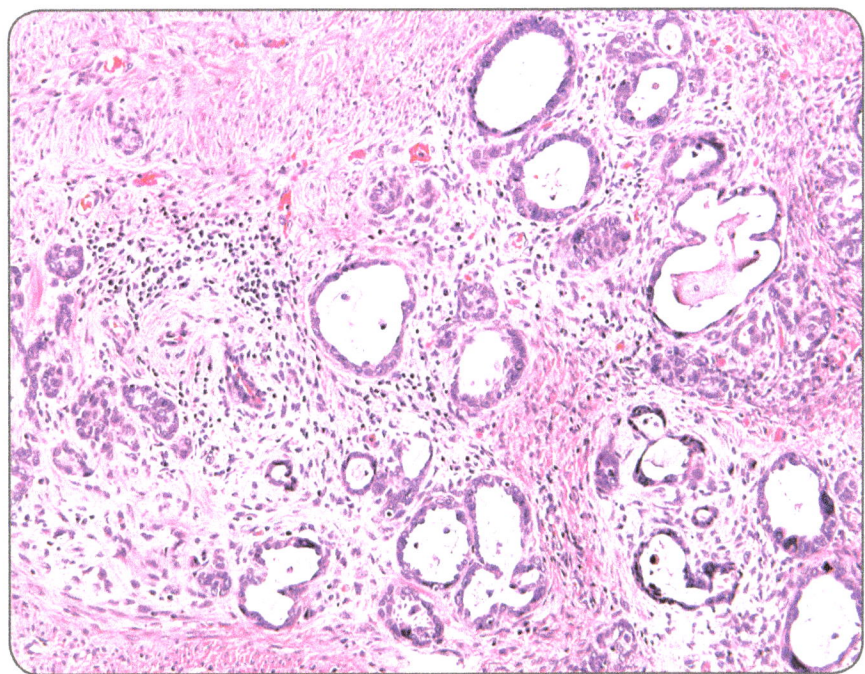

Figure 1.11

Answer: E. Mesonephric adenocarcinoma

Comment: This tumor is a **mesonephric adenocarcinoma** composed of tubular structures lined by flattened cuboidal epithelium. Neoplastic tubules are surrounded by small glandular mesonephric remnants, best seen on the left side of the Figure 1.11. These mesonephric remnants and the tumor cells reacted with the antibody to GATA3, a good marker of both neoplastic and non-neoplastic mesonephric epithelium (*Source:* Roma AA, et al. J Gynecol Pathol. 2015; 34: 480-6).

Q.36 This invasive cervical carcinoma (Figure 1.12) was diagnosed in a 50-year-old woman. It was positive immunohistochemically for p16 and negative for synaptophysin and chromogranin. What is the most likely diagnosis?

A. Papillary squamous cell carcinoma
B. Keratinizing squamous cell carcinoma
C. Small cell neuroendocrine carcinoma
D. Adenosquamous carcinoma
E. Lymphoepithelioma-like carcinoma

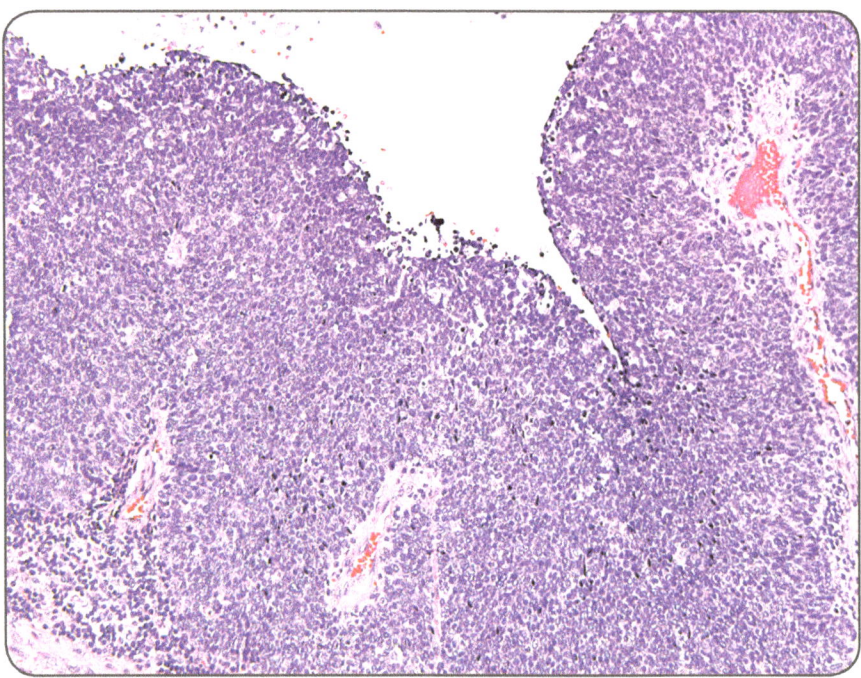

Figure 1.12

Answer: A. Papillary squamous cell carcinoma

Comment: This tumor has fibrovascular cores lined by small blue cells with oval nuclei and scant cytoplasm resembling a thick layer of carcinoma in situ (CIN 3). Human papillomavirus (HPV) is found in approximately one-half of all cases. This rare variant of cervical carcinoma has a tendency to recur or metastasize in 30% of cases. Other variants of invasive squamous carcinoma are as follows: keratinizing, verrucous, warty, basaloid and lymphoepithelioma-like.

Q.37 Which of the following rare cervical tumors has the best prognosis?
  A. Adenoid basal carcinoma
  B. Adenosquamous carcinoma
  C. Adenoid cystic carcinoma
  D. Small cell neuroendocrine tumor
  E. Malignant mixed Müllerian tumor

Answer: A. Adenoid basal carcinoma

Comment: Adenoid basal carcinoma has an excellent prognosis in contrast to other rare tumors listed here, which have bad prognosis.

Q.38 Neuroendocrine tumors of the cervix are most often classified as:
  A. Carcinoid
  B. Atypical carcinoid
  C. Small cell neuroendocrine carcinoma
  D. Large cell neuroendocrine carcinoma
  E. None of the above

Answer: C. Small cell neuroendocrine carcinoma

Comment: **Neuroendocrine tumors** of the cervix are uncommon accounting for less than 2% of all cervical malignant tumors. Small cell neuroendocrine carcinoma (SCNC) is the most common subtype of these tumors. It must be distinguished from small cell squamous cell carcinoma and even more uncommon metastases of SCNC from lung, urinary bladder or pancreas and gastrointestinal tract.

Q.39 This endocervical tumor (Figure 1.13) was immunohistochemically positive for synaptophysin and chromogranin. What is the most likely diagnosis?

    A. Basaloid squamous cell carcinoma
    B. Carcinoid
    C. Small cell neuroendocrine carcinoma
    D. Adenoid basal carcinoma
    E. Adenoid cystic carcinoma

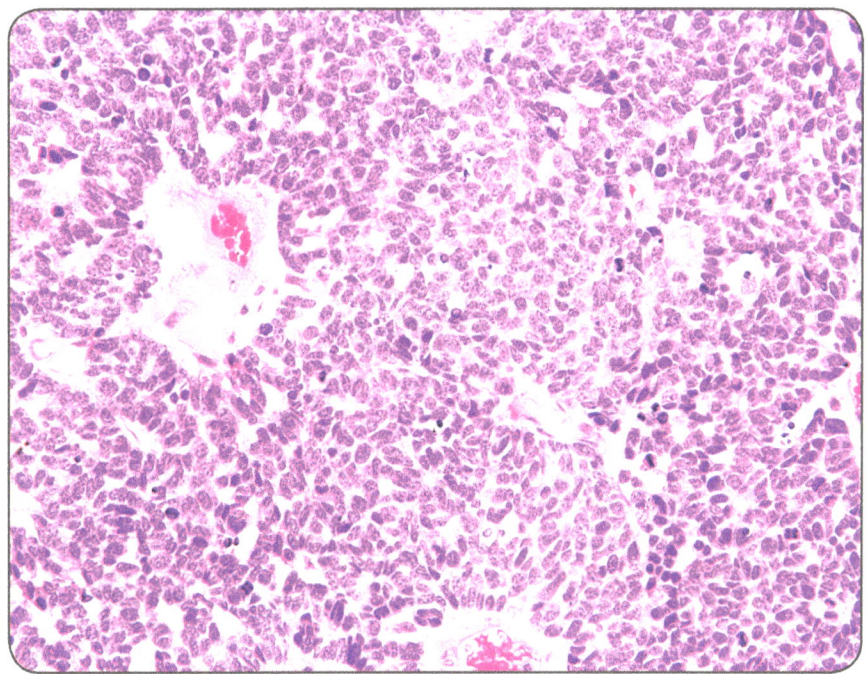

Figure 1.13

Answer: **C. Small cell neuroendocrine carcinoma**

Comment: This small blue cell tumor was shown by immunohistochemistry to be composed of neuroendocrine cells and it has features similar to small cell carcinoma.

Q.40 This endocervical carcinoma (Figure 1.14) was removed from a 55-year-old woman. The tumor cells reacted with PAS, and became unreactive with PAS after diastase digestion. Focally, it was mucicarmine positive. What is the most likely diagnosis?

    A. Squamous cell carcinoma
    B. Clear cell adenosquamous carcinoma
    C. Mesonephric carcinoma
    D. Adenoid basal carcinoma
    E. Adenoid cystic carcinoma

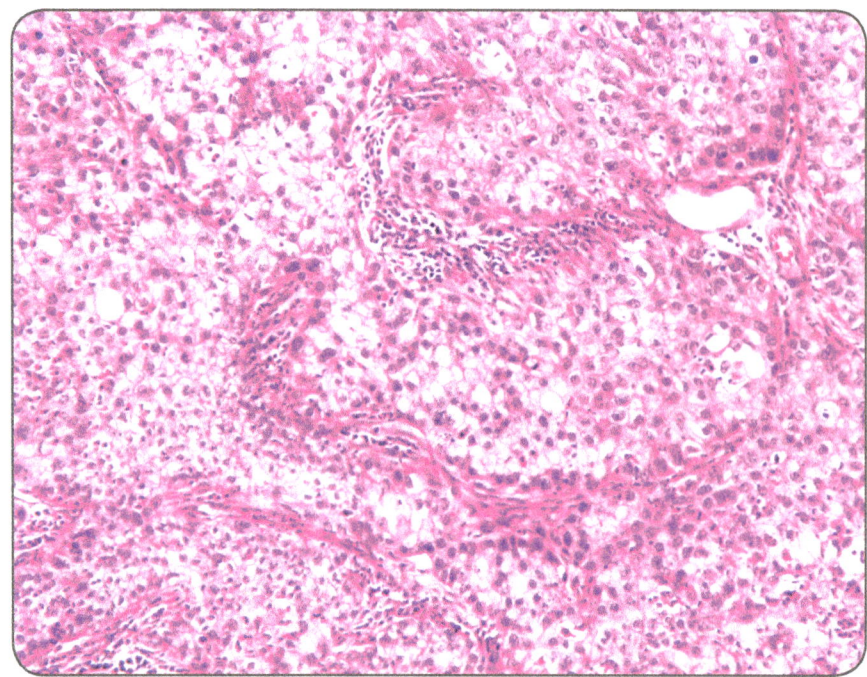

Figure 1.14

Answer: B. Clear cell adenosquamous carcinoma

Comment: **Clear cell adenosquamous carcinoma** is composed predominantly of cells that have clear cytoplasm. The periodic acid–Schiff (PAS) stain combined with diastase predigestion shows that the cells contain large amounts of glycogen. The tumor cells are arranged into sheets with vague attempts of gland formation. The septa contain lymphocytes. All these features are typical of adenosquamous carcinoma, a highly malignant tumor related to HPV 18 infection.

This tumor needs to be distinguished from **clear cell carcinomas**, identical to the clear cell carcinoma of the ovary. This highly malignant tumor consists of clear cells forming solid sheets, or tubulocystic and papillary structures lined by clear and hobnailed cells.

Adenosquamous carcinomas contain foci of keratinized epithelium with keratin pearls but also well-formed glands.

Glassy cell carcinomas are composed of polygonal cells with ground glass pink cytoplasm and prominent cell membranes.

Q.41 What is the most common vaginal malignant tumor in children?

 A. Embryonal rhabdomyosarcoma
 B. Yolk sac tumor
 C. Leiomyosarcoma
 D. Clear cell carcinoma
 E. Squamous cell carcinoma

Answer: A. Embryonal rhabdomyosarcoma

Comment: **Embryonal rhabdomyosarcoma** (*sarcoma botryoides*) is the most common vaginal tumor of childhood. There are not more than reported 100-150 yolk sac tumors of the vagina mostly in children and young women. Leiomyosarcomas are also rare and occur in in older women. Clear cell carcinoma of the cervix and vagina was reported in 20th century in young women born to mothers treated with stilbestrol during pregnancy, but are rare today.

Q.42 What is the most common primary site of tumors that have metastasized to the vagina?
- A. Cervix
- B. Endometrium
- C. Rectum
- D. Ovary
- E. Vulva

Answer: **A. Cervix**

Comment: The most common primary site of metastatic carcinomas in the vagina is cervix, which harbors approximately one-third of all these tumors. The next common site is endometrium accounting for one-fifth of metastatic tumors, followed by the primaries in other organs listed here as possible answers and in that same order of frequency.

Q.43. What is the most likely diagnosis for the endocervical tumor shown in Figure 1.15?
- A. Clear cell carcinoma
- B. Adenoid cystic carcinoma
- C. Adenosquamous carcinoma
- D. Squamous cell carcinoma
- E. Rhabdomyosarcoma

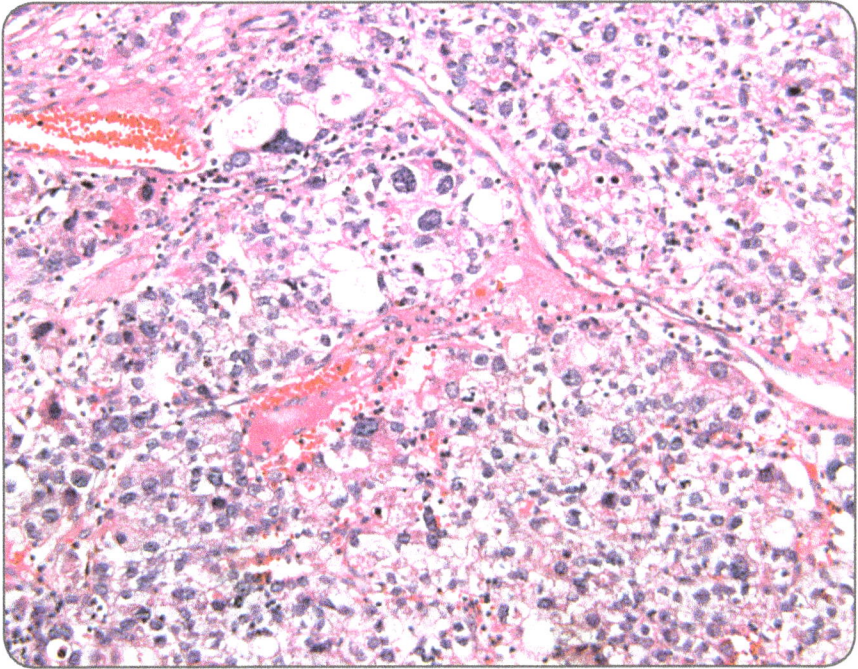

Figure 1.15

Answer: **A. Clear cell carcinoma**

Comment: This malignant tumor is composed of hyperchromatic clear cells arranged in solid sheets. This uncommon endocervical tumor is indistinguishable from **clear cell carcinoma** of the ovary displaying a solid growth pattern.

CHAPTER 2

Uterus

Q.1 All the following statements are true about the lower endometrial segment of the uterus, *except:*
   A. Glands contain nondescript columnar and scattered ciliated cells
   B. Glands have narrow lumens and do not contain endocervical-like mucus secreting cells
   C. Glands show cyclic changes in response to hormonal stimuli
   D. In contrast to fundic endometrium stroma is more fibrotic and the cells have more elongated nuclei
   E. This part of the uterus is also called uterine isthmus

Answer: C. Glands show cyclic changes in response to hormonal stimuli

Comment: The transition from endocervical to endometrial mucosa is gradual. The glands of this transitional zone called **lower uterine segment** or **uterine isthmus** are lined by cells that differ from mucus secreting cells of endocervical glands as well the endometrium proper. These glands do not respond to hormonal stimuli and in contrast to endometrial glands do not show cyclic change corresponding to the proliferative and secretory phase of the menstrual cycle. The glands are lined by nondescript columnar cells and a few scattered ciliated cells. The stroma is more fibrotic than the endometrial stroma.

Q.2 Estrogenic stimulation of endometrium leads to a prominence of which normal endometrial cells?
   A. Secretory cells
   B. Clear cells
   C. Ciliated cells
   D. Basal cells
   E. Endothelial cells in spiral arteries

Answer: C. Ciliated cells

Comment: **Ciliated cells** are most prominent in the endometrial mucosa toward the lower uterine segment and the border zone toward the fallopian tubes in the uterine cornua. However, scattered ciliated cells may be seen anywhere in the surface epithelium of the endometrium proper. **Estrogen** contributes to the prominence of ciliated cells, which appear to multiply and/or assume the ciliated cell phenotype under estrogenic stimulation.

Q.3 Which of the following represent the characteristic early secretory changes in the endometrium?
   A. Apoptosis of surface epithelium
   B. Subnuclear vacuoles in the glands of the stratum spongiosum
   C. Supranuclear vacuoles in the glands of stratum basale
   D. Supranuclear vacuoles in the glands of stratum compactum
   E. Edema of the stroma

Answer: B. Subnuclear vacuoles in the glands of the stratum spongiosum

Comment: **Subnuclear vacuoles** in the glands of the zona compacta or zona spongiosa (which are the two parts of stratum functionale) are early signs of **secretory activity** that begins after ovulation under the influence of progesterone. Subnuclear vacuoles appear approximately 2 days after ovulation. Glands of the basal layer do not respond to progesterone, and the changes in the surface epithelium are relatively minor and do not include apoptosis. Supranuclear vacuoles in the glandular epithelium are seen in the postovulatory secretory endometrium. Edema of the stroma is a feature of mid to late proliferative endometrium. Edema disappears at ovulation to reappear around day 22 of a 28 day cycle.

Q.4 **What is the best diagnosis for the endometrial biopsy shown in Figure 2.1?**
   A. Proliferative endometrium
   B. Mid-secretory endometrium
   C. Menstrual endometrium
   D. Endometrial hyperplasia
   E. Disorderly proliferative endometrium

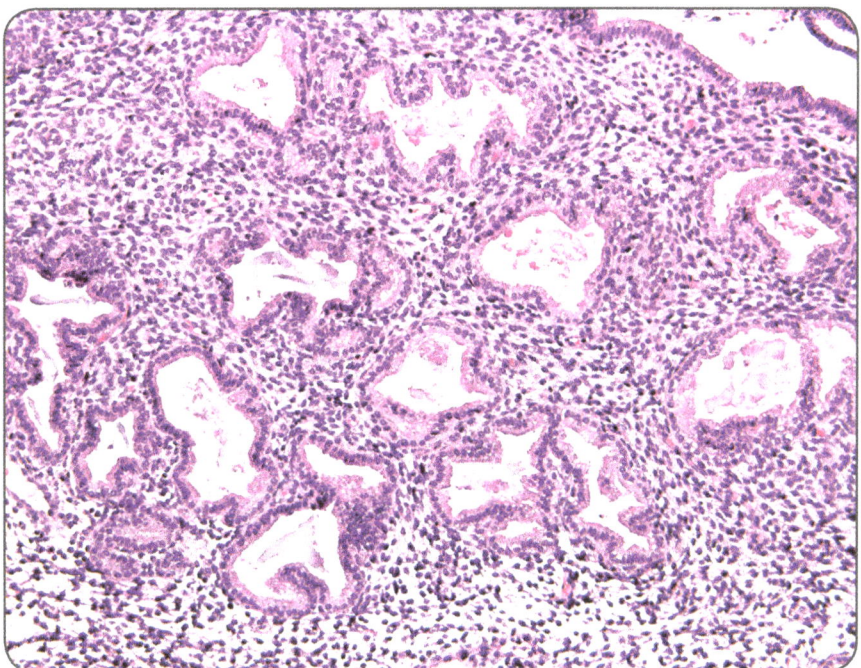

Figure 2.1

Answer: **B. Mid-secretory endometrium**

Comment: The secretory phase of the menstrual cycle can be divided into three stages: Early (postovulatory), mid-secretory, and late secretory. **Early secretory** glands have subnuclear vacuoles, some remaining proliferative glands and stroma that resembles proliferative phase endometrium.

Mid-secretory endometrium (5 to 9 days after ovulation, or day 19 to day 23 of a typical 28 day cycle) is characterized by dilated angular and glands secreting proteinaceous material into their lumens. The stroma is focally edematous and slightly eosinophilic due to the progesterone effect. In the **late secretory** endometrium, there is secretory exhaustion and the glands appear more serrated. Stroma shows predecidual changes, especially around the spiral arteries. Stromal lymphocytes are prominent. Neutrophils appear before the menstrual shedding, which is characterized by stromal breakdown.

Proliferative phase endometrium is composed of small tubular glands widely spaced in a relatively densely cellular stroma. Mitotic figures are present in the stroma and the glands.

Menstrual endometrium is characterized by collapsed glands which still may show some signs of secretion. Condensed "stromal blue balls" are prominent. Stromal breakdown is marked by areas of necrosis, infiltrates of neutrophils, and hemorrhage.

Q.5 Which of the following statements is true about the predecidual changes?

A. Predecidual change occurs within hours after ovulation
B. Predecidual change occurs only 2-3 days prior to menstruation
C. Predecidual change occurs only in the presence of a fertilized ovum
D. Predecidual change is mediated by progesterone
E. Predecidual change begins first in stratum basale

Answer: D. Predecidual change is mediated by progesterone

Comment: **Predecidual change** results from the effects of progesterone on stromal cells of the stratum functionale, and it is not seen in stratum basale. Even the deep layers of stratum spongiosum do not undergo decidualization. Decidua appears around the day 22 of a 28 day cycle, usually around the spiral arteries, and its appearance is not related to pregnancy or impending menstruation. Oral contraceptives and exogenous progesterone may induce predecidual reaction. Foci of endometriosis also may show signs of decidualization.

Q.6 When during a typical 28 day menstrual cycle does intraluminal secretion appear in the endometrial glands?

A. Day 15
B. Day 16
C. Days 19-21
D. Days 23-24
E. Days 25-27

Answer: C. Days 19-21

Comment: **Mid-secretory endometrial glands** on days 19-21 contain **secretory material**. Toward the end of the menstrual cycle they show "secretory exhaustion" assuming a serrated luminal ("saw-toothed") appearance.

Q.7 What are the CD 163 positive cells normally found immunohistochemically in the endometrium?

A. B-lymphocytes
B. Macrophages
C. T-helper lymphocytes
D. Cytotoxic T lymphocytes
E. Natural killer cells

Answer: B. Macrophages

Comment: **CD 163**, a glycoprotein that belongs to the scavenger receptor of the cysteine-rich superfamily, is a marker of **macrophages and monocytes**. These cells are normally present in the endometrium, regulating the immune response. CD163 is important for clearing haptoglobin-hemoglobin complexes from blood and tissues.

Q.8 Aggregates of stromal cells ("blue balls") juxtaposed to strips of glandular cells that have an eosinophilic cytoplasm are typical of which days of a normal 28 day menstrual cycle?

A. Days 10-12
B. Days 18-20
C. Days 21-23
D. Day 24-25
E. Days 1-3 (menstruation)

Answer: E. Day 1-3 (menstruation)

Comment: Fragmentation and breakdown of endometrium with formation of blue balls composed of stromal cells and strips of eosinophilic glandular cells are typical of **menstrual endometrium**. Sometimes, the glandular cells show nests of so called "**papillary syncytial metaplasia**". The stroma is **decidualized** and infiltrated with **neutrophils**.

Q.9 What is the best diagnosis for the changes seen in the endometrial currettings shown in Figure 2.2.?
   A. Proliferative endometrium
   B. Mid-secretory endometrium
   C. Menstrual endometrium
   D. Pregnancy-related changes
   E. Changes related to oral contraceptives

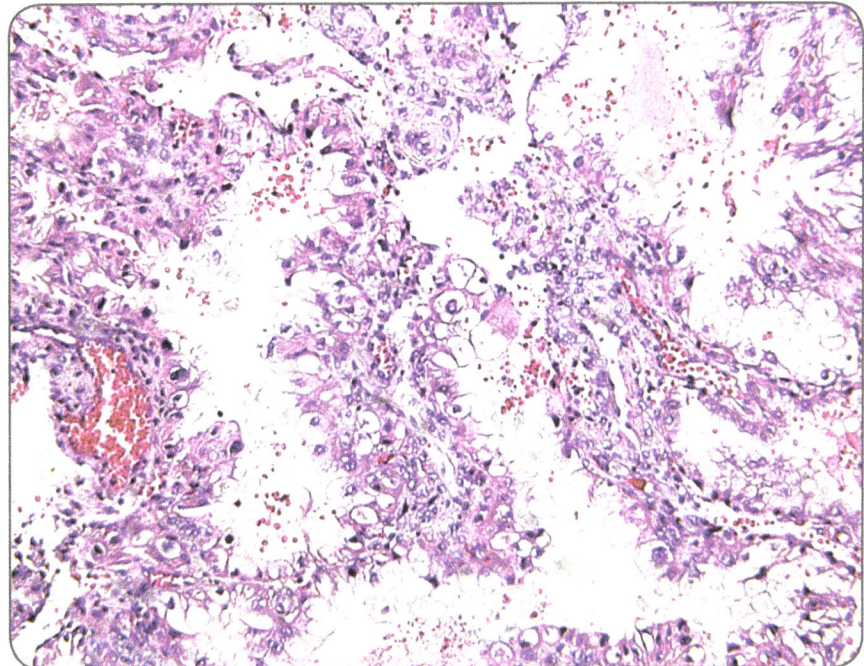

Figure 2.2

Answer: D. Pregnancy-related changes

Comment: The endometrial glands in this specimen are lined by large stratified cells that have clear cytoplasm and hyperchromatic nuclei.

Q.10 Arias-Stella reaction of pregnancy may be found in all the following sites or lesions, *except:*
   A. Endometrium of the uterine cornua
   B. Endocervix
   C. Fallopian tubes
   D. Adenomyosis of the myometrium
   E. Endometriosis of the ovary

Answer: D. Adenomyosis of the myometrium

Comment: **Arias-Stella reaction of pregnancy** is characterized by the appearance of enlarged hyperchromatic nuclei in clear "hypersecretory" endometrial glands. Some cells even appear hobnail-like, and may show intranuclear inclusions. This reaction usually involves the endometrium but during the pregnancy it may be seen in the endocervix, fallopian tubes, and even in foci of endometriosis. It does not involve adenomyosis, which is composed of hormone insensitive glands resembling the normal stratum basale of the uterus.

Q.11 Which cells are more numerous in the endometrium of pregnant than non-pregnant women?
- A. B-lymphocytes
- B. Plasma cells
- C. T-helper lymphocytes
- D. Cytotoxic T lymphocytes
- E. Natural killer (NK) cells

Answer: **E. Natural killer (NK) cells**

Comment: The number of **natural killer (NK)** cells gradually will increase in the endometrium after implantation. By mid-pregnancy NK cells may account for 70% of all stromal lymphocytes. It has been proposed that NK cells play an important role in infertility, but that hypothesis has not been confirmed in well-controlled studies. The number of **B lymphocytes** is low in the normal endometrium, and it does not increase during pregnancy. **Plasma cells** are also sparse, and some authorities believe that the normal endometrium does not contain any plasma cells at all. **T lymphocytes** vary in number during pregnancy. Their numbers may decrease in some pregnant uteri, but as a rule their numbers do not increase during pregnancy.

Q.12 All the following are typical of postmenopausal atrophy of the endometrium, *except:*
- A. Low cuboidal surface epithelium
- B. Cystic change of glands
- C. Accumulation of serous fluid in the glandular lumen
- D. Fibrosis of the stroma
- E. Infiltrates of neutrophils in the stroma

Answer: **E. Infiltrates of neutrophils in the stroma**

Comment: **Atrophic endometrium of postmenopausal women** is thin and composed of nondescript glands lined by low cuboidal or flattened nondescript epithelium. Atrophic glands cannot be classified as either proliferative or secretory, and are occasionally called "inactive". They do not show any signs of acute inflammation. Accordingly, neutrophils are not found in atrophic endometria, unless there is infection. Also there is no secretory activity, although some cystically dilated glands may contain proteinaceous material. This material may represent a transudate of serum or hormone-independent residual basal secretion of these atrophic glands. Stroma appears fibrotic.

Q.13 Which of the following tissues represent an unusual and unexpected finding in endometrial curettings that should be reported to the gynecologist submitting the tissue for histopathologic examination?
- A. Endocervical tissue
- B. Exocervical squamous epithelium
- C. Brain tissue
- D. Bone and cartilage
- E. Mature fat tissue

Answer: **E. Mature fat tissue**

Comment: Finding of **mature fat tissue** in the endometrial **curettings** should be reported because it may be omental fat that has been reached through the perforated uterine wall. Cervical and exocervical tissues are commonly included in endometrial biopsies. Brain, cartilage or bone found in the curetting are most often of fetal origin, and are usually combined with decidua and other endometrial changes induced by pregnancy.

Q.14 All the following are microscopic features of anovulatory endometrial shedding, *except:*
- **A.** Proliferative endometrial glands
- **B.** Focal cystic dilatation and branching of glands
- **C.** Ciliated cells and cell with eosinophilic cytoplasm in some glands
- **D.** Fibrin thrombi in small endometrial vessels
- **E.** Focal predecidual reaction of the stroma

Answer: **E. Focal predecidual reaction of the stroma**

Comment: **Anovulatory shedding** differs from the menstrual shedding of the endometrium in one major respect: Without ovulation there is no progesterone effect and the endometrium remains in an extended proliferative phase. Thus, the glands show no signs of secretion or secretory exhaustion and the stroma shows no decidualization. Secondary changes such as cystic dilatation or branching of glands, some of which are lined by cells with cilia or cells with eosinophilic cytoplasm, reflect disorderly proliferation and/or prolonged estrogen stimulation. Fibrin thrombi may be also found. They help distinguishing anovulatory from menstrual shedding. Fibrin thrombi are namely not found in menstrual shedding because of physiological fibrinolysis in the menstruating uterus.

Q.15 What is the best diagnosis for the endometrial biopsy shown in Figure 2.3?
- **A.** Proliferative endometrium
- **B.** Mid-secretory endometrium
- **C.** Menstrual endometrium
- **D.** Endometrial hyperplasia without atypia
- **E.** Disordered proliferative endometrium

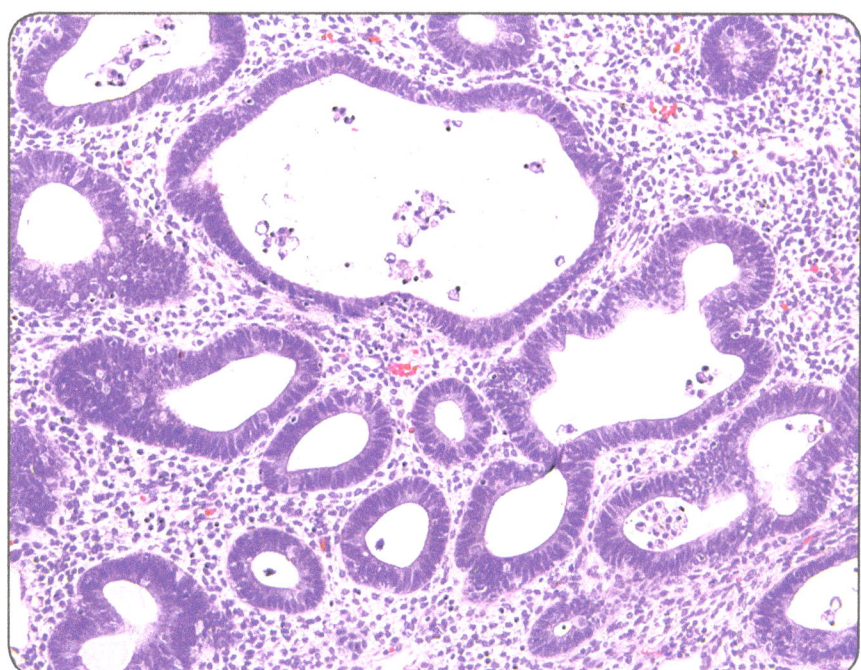

Figure 2.3

Answer: E. Disordered proliferative endometrium

Comment: This endometrial biopsy shows changes lying in between normal proliferative endometrium and simple hyperplasia, commonly diagnosed as **disordered proliferative endometrium.** These changes include focally cystic dilatation of glands lined by proliferative epithelium and glands that show additional periodic "waste-like" narrowing. Scattered normal small tubular proliferative glands also may be seen. The stroma is dense and focally edematous. There is some focal crowding of glands, but overall the ratio of stroma to glands is within the normal range. These endometrial changes are typical of anovulatory cycles, most often encountered in perimenopausal women.

Q.16 What are the changes seen in the endometrial biopsy of most women who have been taking progesterone containing contraceptive pills for extended periods of time?
- A. Atrophy of glands and atrophy of stroma
- B. Atrophy of glands and decidualization of stroma
- C. Secretory glands, variable changes in the stroma
- D. Secretory glands and decidualization of stroma
- E. Hyperplasia of glands and edema of stroma

Answer: B. Atrophy of glands and decidualization of stroma

Comment: In most women taking progesteronic contraceptives there is atrophy of glands and decidualization of the stroma. In very long users, the entire endometrium atrophies and resembles normal postmenopausal endometrium.

Q.17 What is the best diagnosis for the endometrial biopsy shown in Figure 2.4?
- A. Proliferative endometrium
- B. Mid-secretory endometrium
- C. Menstrual endometrium
- D. Pregnancy-related changes
- E. Changes related to oral contraceptives

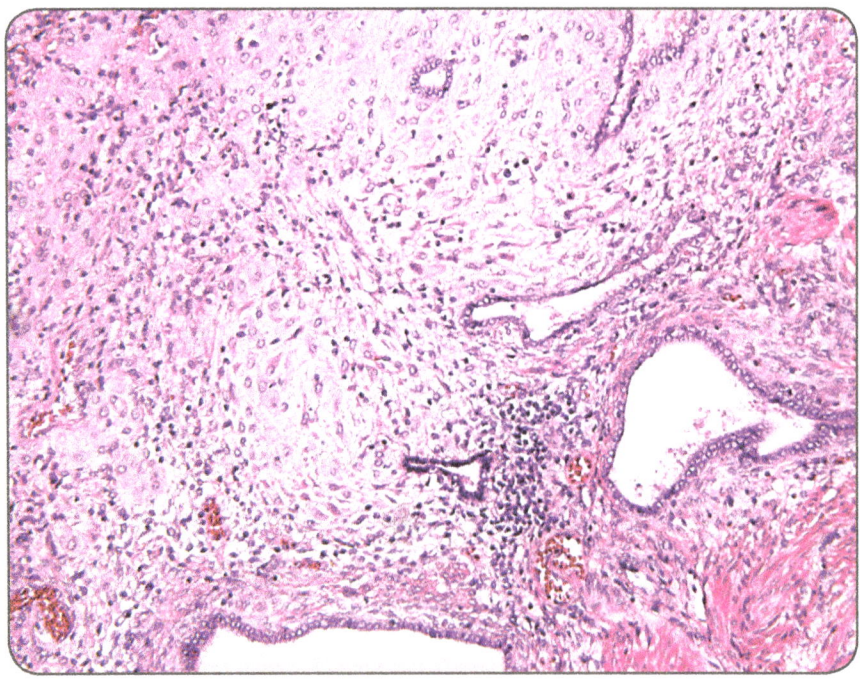

Figure 2.4

Answer: E. Changes related to oral contraceptives

Comment: Figure 2.4 shows stratum basale and myometrial smooth muscle cells on the right hand side and decidualized stroma of the stratum functionale containing small atrophic glands on the left hand side. These changes are induced by **oral contraceptives** and are colloquially called "**pill endometrium**".

Q.18 All the following are microscopic features of nonspecific chronic endometritis, *except:*
   A. Edema
   B. Infiltrates of plasma cells and lymphocytes
   C. Vascular ectasia
   D. Glandular hyperplasia
   E. Breakdown and fragmentation of stroma

Answer: D. Glandular hyperplasia

Comment: **Chronic endometritis** is characterized by uneven and patchy distribution of edema and inflammatory cells, which by definition must include prominent plasma cells. Lymphoid tissue may form prominent follicles with germinal centers. Chlamydial infection and gonorrhea are accompanied by additional infiltrates of neutrophils in the superficial part of endometrium.

Chronic inflammation is accompanied by a loss of estrogen and progesterone receptors on glandular cell. Accordingly, the glands do not show features of either proliferative or secretory endometrium. There is no evidence of hyperplasia. Instead, glands appear "inactive" or "weakly proliferative" or may be "asynchronous" (out of phase or mixed proliferative and secretory). Such endometrium cannot be dated properly. Metaplasia, which is most often eosinophilic or squamous, may be present. Stroma contains spindle cells and may show signs of breakdown. Vascular ectasia is also often seen.

Q.19 Which of the following represents the most common cause of purulent chronic endometritis in women using intrauterine contraceptive devices for more than 3 years?
   A. *Chlamydia trachomatis*
   B. *Mycoplasma genitalium*
   C. *Mycobacterium kansasii*
   D. *Ureaplasma urealyticum*
   E. *Actinomyces israelii*

Answer: E. *Actinomyces israelii*

Comment: *A. israelii* is a Gram positive filamentous pathogen forming "sulfur granules" in the neutrophil-rich exudate that is characteristically present in this chronic **purulent infection**. *Actinomyces sp.* can be impregnated with methenamine silver according to Gomori. Stroma usually shows signs of decidualization and the glands are atrophic and inactive.

Q.20 What is the most likely cause of endometritis shown in Figure 2.5?
   A. *Chlamydia trachomatis*
   B. *Mycoplasma genitalium*
   C. *Mycobacterium kansasii*
   D. *Ureaplasma urealyticum*
   E. *Actinomyces israelii*

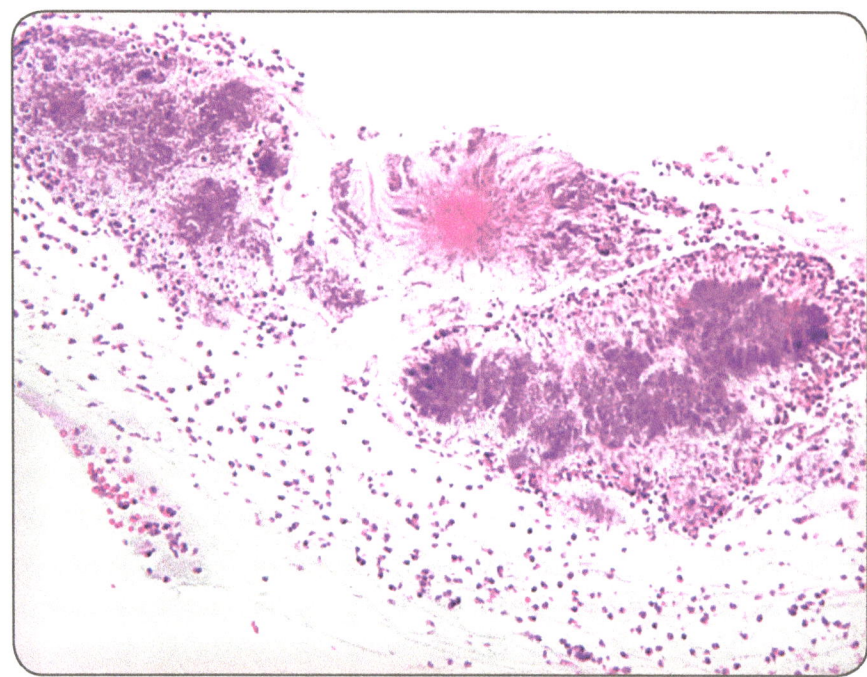

Figure 2.5

Answer: E. *Actinomyces israelii*

Comment: Figure 2.5 shows aggregates of radiating filaments of **Actinomyces israelii**. Larger aggregates may be seen on gross examination floating in the pus and thus corresponding to the so called sulfur granules. The sample was obtained from a woman who had endometritis related to an intrauterine contraceptive device. The diagnosis was confirmed by bacteriologic cultures under anaerobic conditions.

Q.21 Xanthogranulomatous endometritis is characterized by all the following, *except:*

    A. Foamy macrophages
    B. Siderophages with brown cytoplasmic hemosiderin granules
    C. Other chronic and acute inflammatory cells besides macrophages
    D. Granulomas
    E. Fibrosis or calcification

Answer: D. Granulomas

Comment: **Xanthogranulomatous endometritis**, also known as histiocytic chronic endometritis may be caused by radiation but is most often a disease of unknown etiology. The endometrium does not contain **granulomas**, which are usually found in tuberculosis, sarcoidosis, some viral infections, and even in actinomycosis. Granulomas are also part of foreign body giant cell reactions; foreign material can be often seen in the cytoplasm of multinucleated giant cells.

Q.22 Chronic nonspecific endometritis may accompany other endometrial diseases. These anatomic or "structural abnormality related" forms of chronic non-suppurative endometritis include all the following, *except:*
   A. Endometrial polyps
   B. Submucosal leiomyoma
   C. Endometrial carcinoma
   D. Prolapse of the uterus
   E. Postpartum sepsis

Answer: **E. Postpartum sepsis**

Comment: **Chronic nonspecific inflammation** is commonly seen in endometrial and endocervical polyps and endometrium compressed, infiltrated or irritated by tumors.
   Prolapsed uterus usually shows signs of chronic cervicitis which may spread into the uterine cavity.
   Postpartum sepsis may be caused by pyogenic bacteria, or retained placental tissue. It is typically acute and suppurative and microscopically marked by infiltrates of neutrophils. It responds well to antibiotics and surgical evacuation of the causative material form in the uterine cavity.

Q.23 Which of the following is typically found in most if not all endometrial polyps?
   A. Acute inflammation
   B. Granulomas
   C. Cycling endometrium
   D. Loose edematous stroma
   E. Thick-walled blood vessels

Answer: **E. Thick-walled blood vessels**

Comment: Three microscopic findings typically seen in most **endometrial polyps** include:
- **Thick-walled blood vessels**
- **Stroma** that is uniformly cellular ("blue") or fibrotic
- **Dilated glands** that are often irregularly shaped.

   For confident diagnosis of polyps, at least two of these three elements should be identified. Infarcted, twisted or irritated polyps may show chronic inflammation which however is not seen in all polyps. Acute inflammation may be seen in ulcerated or infected polyps, but is not a constant feature either. The epithelial surface composed of irregularly shaped endometrial glands is usually inactive and non-cycling. In some cases, the endometrium of the polyps may show focal secretory changes but if present it is usually lagging in phase, a few days behind the rest of the uterine epithelium.

Q.24 What is the best diagnosis for the endometrial lesion shown in Figure 2.6?
   A. Endometrial polyp
   B. Microglandular hyperplasia
   C. Endometrial atrophy
   D. Endometrial hyperplasia without atypia
   E. Adenomyoma, endometrioid type

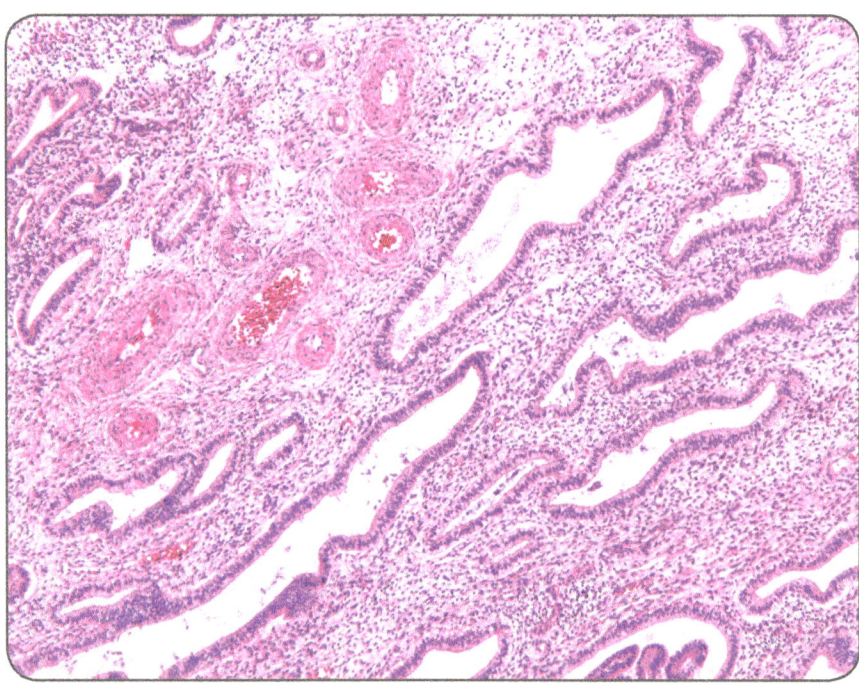

Figure 2.6

Answer: **A. Endometrial polyp**

Comment: Figure 2.6 shows the typical features of an endometrial polyp: Thick-walled blood vessel and dilated glands surrounded by a densely cellular stroma.

Microglandular hyperplasia, characterized by crowding of small but non-neoplastic glands occurs in the endocervix and not in the endometrium.

Endometrial atrophy is characterized by small dilated glands lined by flattened epithelium.

Endometrial hyperplasia shows numerous hyperplastic glands surrounded by scant stroma.

Adenomyoma, endometrioid type, consists of nests of endometrioid glands with a thin rim of endometrial stroma surrounded by smooth muscle cells, which represent the principal cellular component of these tumors.

Q.25 On gross examination endometrial polyps may have the following forms, *except*:
  A. Wart-like protuberance
  B. Finger-like elongated mass sticking into the uterine cavity
  C. Pedunculated mass with a stalk linking it to endometrial surface
  D. Smooth-surfaced mass filling the uterine cavity
  E. Deep mucosal ulceration

Answer: **E. Deep mucosal ulceration**

Comment: Common to all **polyps** is that they all **protrude from the surface** of the endometrium into the uterine cavity. Polyps do not present as ulcerations, even though their surface may be focally eroded or even ulcerated.

Q.26 Which of the following changes is most often seen in postmenopausal ("senile") endometrial polyps?
  A. Papillary proliferation
  B. Squamous metaplasia
  C. Flattened epithelium lining cystic glands often filled with serous fluid
  D. Arias-Stella phenomenon
  E. Hobnail metaplasia

Answer: C. Flattened epithelium lining cystic glands often filled with serous fluid

Comment: **Cystic glands** lined by thin epithelium may be very prominent in postmenopausal endometrial polyps, reflecting the **atrophy** of the entire endometrium.
   Papillary proliferation on the surface of some polyps can occur at any age but is uncommon. If present, it should not be confused with neoplasia.
   Squamous metaplasia is a reparative process which may be seen on the surface of polyps at any age.
   Arias-Stella phenomenon is seen in pregnancy and is not seen in postmenopausal polyps.
   Hobnail metaplasia occurs in response to injury and it is usually seen on the surface of infarcted or mechanically injured polyps.

Q.27 Which of the following forms of metaplasia of endometrium consists of foci of immature squamous epithelium?
   A. Papillary syncytial metaplasia
   B. Tubal metaplasia
   C. Eosinophilic metaplasia
   D. Morular metaplasia
   E. Hobnail metaplasia

Answer: D. Morular metaplasia

Comment: **Morular metaplasia** consist of small balls or immature squamous epithelium. These foci may contain areas of central necrosis but there is no proliferative activity. Other forms of metaplasia mentioned in this question do not contain squamous cells.
   Papillary syncytial metaplasia usually involves the superficial epithelium. It consists of cells with eosinophilic cytoplasm and indistinct borders forming pseudopapillae without connective tissue cores. Their nuclei are often smudged. This change is typically seen in association with stromal breakdown at the time of menstruation or anovulatory bleeding.
   Tubal metaplasia is marked by the appearance of numerous ciliated cells and other tubal cells, often formed in response to excessive continuous estrogenic stimulation.
   Eosinophilic metaplasia is marked by the formation of oncocytes, i.e. cuboidal and even cylindrical cells that contain numerous mitochondria in their cytoplasm.
   Hobnail metaplasia is marked by the appearance of cells that have bulging apical poles and often apically displaced nuclei with mild hyperchromasia.

Q.28 All of the following are acceptable terms for the WHO recommended diagnosis of "endometrial hyperplasia without atypia", *except:*
   A. Simple cystic hyperplasia
   B. Simple endometrial hyperplasia without atypia
   C. Simple non-atypical endometrial hyperplasia
   D. Complex non-atypical endometrial hyperplasia
   E. Complex endometrial hyperplasia without atypia

Answer: A. Simple cystic hyperplasia

Comment: WHO committee has recommended a **two-tiered classification** which includes **hyperplasia without atypia** and **atypical hyperplasia**. This classification has replaced the older three tiered classification that also included simple cystic hyperplasia. Endometrium showing focal cystic changes of regularly distributed proliferating glands surrounded by well-developed dense stroma is not considered to be hyperplastic; it is usually signed out as **disordered proliferative endometrium**. It should be noted that the official WHO diagnosis does not contain the terms "simple" or "complex" that were part of previous classifications. Nevertheless, the WHO committee acknowledged that these qualifiers are still used in practice by many pathologists. Accordingly these terms would be acceptable tacitly, as long as the determinants "non-atypical" or "without atypia" are included in the diagnosis.

Q.29 What is the best diagnosis for the endometrial biopsy shown in Figure 2.7?

    A. Disordered proliferative endometrium
    B. Chronic endometritis
    C. Endometrial polyp
    D. Endometrial hyperplasia without atypia
    E. Atypical endometrial hyperplasia

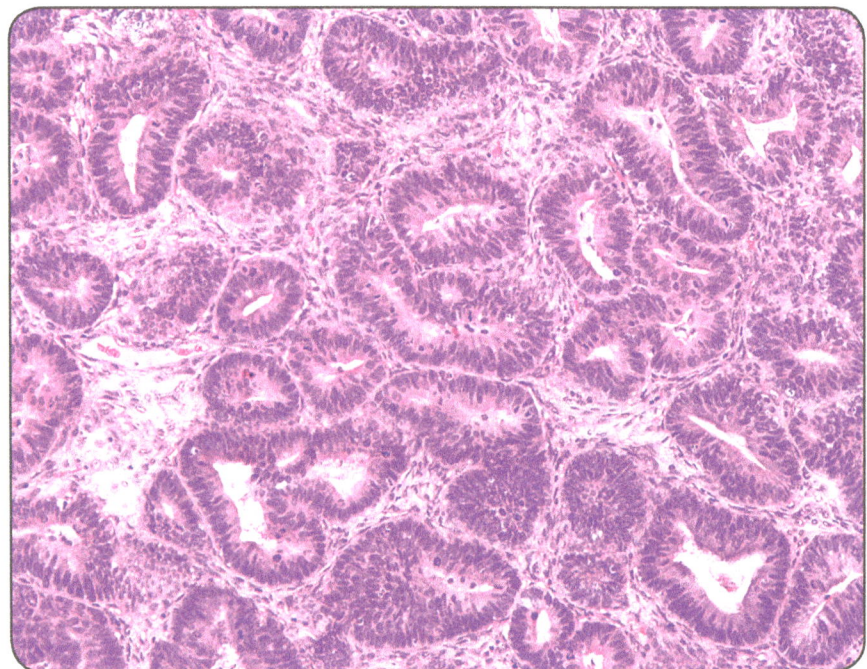

Figure 2.7

Answer: D. Endometrial hyperplasia without atypia

Comment: Figure 2.7 shows typical features of **endometrial hyperplasia without atypia**.
These changes include crowding of the glands, which are lined by columnar epithelium showing relatively uniform stratification of their elongated nuclei. Reduced amounts of stroma accompanied by glandular hyperplasia account for an increased gland to stroma ratio.

Q.30 All the following are typical feature of endometrial hyperplasia without atypia, *except:*

    A. Crowding of glands that may show some focal branching and dilatation
    B. Increased ratio of glands to stroma
    C. Cells lining the glands are columnar with cigar-shaped nuclei
    D. Rounding of nuclei and loss of cell polarity
    E. Focal hemorrhage and stromal breakdown

Answer: D. Rounding of nuclei and loss of cell polarity

Comment: **Endometrial hyperplasia without atypia** includes several characteristic microscopic findings such as: variable crowding of glands that show some focal branching and dilatation; increased ratio of glands to stroma due to a reduced amount of periglandular stroma; columnar cells lining the glands and showing stratification of their cigar-shaped nuclei and mitotic figures.
Focal hemorrhage and stromal breakdown are common. Rounding of nuclei and loss of cell polarity are signs of atypia.

Q.31 Which one of the following terms is the currently WHO recommended synonym for endometrial atypical hyperplasia?
   A. Complex endometrial hyperplasia with atypia
   B. Complex atypical endometrial hyperplasia
   C. Simple atypical hyperplasia
   D. Simple hyperplasia with atypia
   E. Endometrial intraepithelial neoplasia (EIN)

Answer: **E. Endometrial intraepithelial neoplasia (EIN)**

Comment: The contributors to the WHO classification of Tumors of the Female Reproductive Organs (2014) recommend the term **Atypical hyperplasia/Endometrioid intraepithelial neoplasia (EIN)** with a slash between these two terms. It is also known as "endometrial intraepithelial carcinoma", but the use of this term is not encouraged. Other diagnostic terms listed here are included in the WHO "blue book" as acceptable for historical reasons. It is worth a notice that the terms "complex" and "simple" are not included in the WHO designation.

Q.32 All the following are typical feature of atypical endometrial hyperplasia, *except:*
   A. Crowding of cytologically altered glands
   B. Increased ratio of glands to stroma
   C. Villoglandular growth pattern
   D. Loss of polarity of cells lining the glands
   E. Enlargement of nuclei which are round and have nucleoli

Answer: **C. Villoglandular growth pattern**

Comment: Crowding of cytologically altered glands is the defining feature of **endometrial hyperplasia with atypia/EIN**. The size of such crowded groups is important! It should measure at least 1 mm or more. Atypical endometrial hyperplasia resembles endometrial hyperplasia without atypia: Both lesions are composed of crowded glands and there is an increased ratio of glands to stroma, due to scarcity of stroma between the grouped glands. In contrast to the endometrial hyperplasia without atypia, atypical hyperplasia shows a loss of polarity of cells lining the glands. The nuclei of atypical cells are enlarged, rounded and often have nucleoli. **Villoglandular growth** pattern is not a feature of atypical hyperplasia and should be taken as evidence of malignancy, supporting the diagnosis of endometrioid endometrial carcinoma. Stromal invasion, presenting as "back-to-back" or cribriform growth of glands is yet another sign that the atypical hyperplasia has progressed to carcinoma. Readers interested in practicing their diagnostic skill are advised to visit the website *www.endometrium.org.*

Q.33 What is the best diagnosis for the endometrial lesion shown in Figure 2.8?
   A. Disordered proliferative endometrium
   B. Endometrial polyp
   C. Endometrial hyperplasia without atypia
   D. Endometrial hyperplasia with atypia/EIN
   E. Endometrioid adenocarcinoma arising in endometrial hyperplasia with atypia

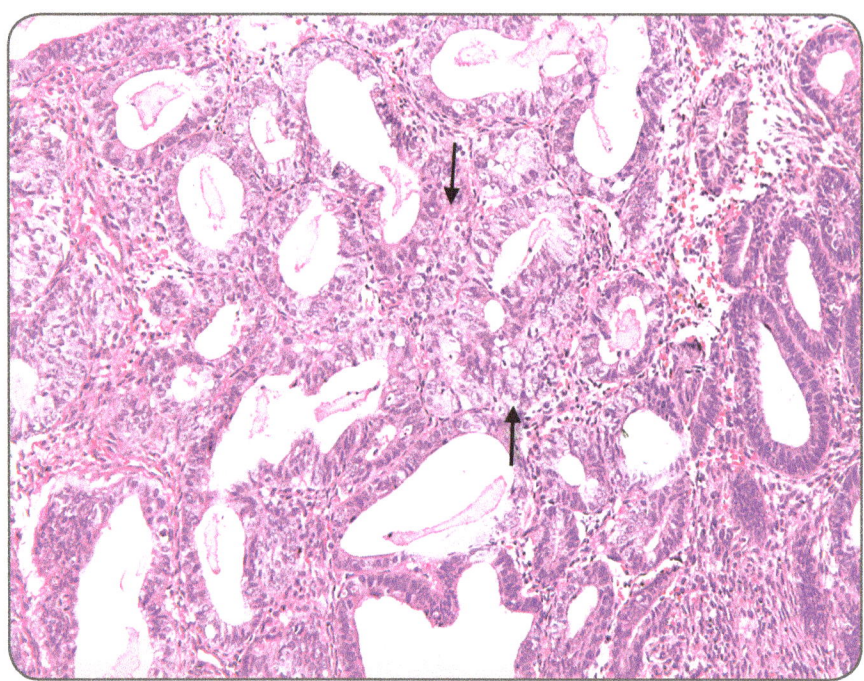

Figure 2.8

Answer: E. Endometrioid adenocarcinoma arising in endometrial hyperplasia with atypia

Comment: The bulk of the lesion consists of **endometrial hyperplasia with atypia.** The enlarged vesicular nuclei of this lesion should be compared with the small dark nuclei of normal endometrial glands along the right hand side border of the figures. In the midfield one can see cribriform glands within glands of **adenocarcinoma** that has evolved in the hyperplastic endometrium (arrows).

Q.34 Which form of metaplasia may occur in atypical endometrial hyperplasia/EIN?
- A. Mucinous
- B. Secretory
- C. Morular
- D. Tubal
- E. All of the above

Answer: E. All of the above

Comment: **Any form of metaplasia** can be seen focally in atypical endometrial hyperplasia and even in adjacent normal glands. Morular balls, which may be quite prominent should not be included in the measurement of the size of hyperplastic areas.

Q.35 All the following increase the risk for the occurrence of atypical endometrial hyperplasia/EIN, *except:*
- A. Obesity
- B. Polycystic ovary syndrome
- C. Prolonged use of oral contraceptives
- D. Hormonal therapy with estrogen without progesterone
- E. Granulosa cell tumors of the ovary

Answer: C. Prolonged use of oral contraceptives

Comment: **Risk factors for atypical endometrial hyperplasia** are the same as those for endometrial adenocarcinoma, and include the well-known causes of excessive estrogenic stimulation of the endometrium, including the following:
- Obesity (peripheral generation of estrogen in fat tissue)
- Exogenous estrogen therapy
- Insulin resistance, diabetes mellitus type II, metabolic syndrome
- Hyperestrinism of the polycystic ovary syndrome (PCOS)
- Estrogen producing tumors of the ovary, such as granulosa or theca cell tumors.

Oral contraceptives reduce significantly the incidence of endometrial hyperplasia and endometrial carcinoma. Estrogen-related endometrioid carcinomas, classified as type I endometrial adenocarcinomas, account for over 80% or all endometrial malignant tumors.

Q.36 Expressed in percentage, how many cases of endometrial hyperplasia without atypia will regresses spontaneously?
- A. 3%
- B. 80%
- C. 20%
- D. 40%
- E. None

Answer: **B. 80%**

Comment: About 80% of the simple and complex endometrial hyperplasia without atypia regresses spontaneously. However, about 30% of the complex hyperplasia with atypia progresses to endometrioid carcinoma.

Q.37 Percentagewise, how many women diagnosed to have atypical hyperplasia/EIN on biopsy will have endometrial carcinoma on subsequent hysterectomy performed within 1 year of diagnosis?
- A. Less than 5%
- B. Less than 20%
- C. 25–30%
- D. 50%
- E. 75–80%

Answer: **C. 25–30%**

Comment: Several studies have come up with the same results indicating that one-forth to one-third of all women with the biopsy diagnosis of **atypical hyperplasia/EIN** will prove to have **endometrial carcinoma** either at the time of biopsy or during the follow-up period of 1 year. Treatment of these women with **progesterone** may reduce the incidence of such carcinomas.

Q.38 Following a biopsy diagnosis of endometrial hyperplasia without atypia, how many of these women (expressed in percentages) will develop endometrioid carcinoma over a 20 year period?
- A. 5%
- B. 20%
- C. 30%
- D. 50%
- E. 66%

Answer: **A. 5%**

Comment: Women with endometrial hyperplasia without atypia are at a **slightly increased risk** for **endometrial carcinoma**, but overall such risk is still very low (approximately 5% at 20 years).

Q.39 Atypical endometrial hyperplasia /EIN is usually localized to a portion of the endometrium but in some cases it may be widespread involving the entire uterine cavity. Expressed in percentage, how many cases of atypical endometrial hyperplasia/EIN occur in such a "non-localized" form?

  A. Less than 5%
  B. 20%
  C. 40%
  D. 60%
  E. 75%

Answer: B. 20%

Comment: Two important pathologic variants of atypical endometrial hyperplasia/EIN are its **diffuse variant** which occurs in about 20% of cases, and the localized type that occurs in **endometrial polyps** (30%).
It should be noted that atypical endometrial hyperplasia/EIN can also involve adenomyosis, and in that case it should not be misinterpreted as invasive endometrioid adenocarcinoma.

Q.40 Which form of endometrial cancer occurs in women afflicted by hereditary nonpolyposis colon cancer with MLH1 inactivation?

  A. Endometrioid carcinoma
  B. Serous carcinoma
  C. Clear cell carcinomas
  D. Squamous cell carcinoma
  E. Undifferentiated carcinoma

Answer: A. Endometrioid carcinoma

Comment: **Hereditary nonpolyposis colorectal cancer (HNPCC)** with **MLH1** (MutL homolog 1) inactivation may be associated with endometrial carcinoma. It is a relatively rare cause of hereditary endometrial carcinoma, accounting for less than 10% of these tumors. Most of these tumors were classified as endometrioid carcinomas.

Q.41 All the following variants of endometrioid carcinoma are recognized by the experts of WHO and included as such in the latest WHO "blue book", *except*:

  A. Villoglandular
  B. Secretory
  C. Mucinous
  D. With squamous differentiation
  E. Papillary

Answer: E. Papillary

Comment: Endometrioid carcinoma of the usual type is defined in the WHO "blue book" as "glandular neoplasm displaying an acinar, papillary or partly solid configuration". It has several variants which have separate ICD-O codes. Even if you are not using these numerical codes, the descriptors for these variants deserve to be included in the diagnosis for prognostic reasons. Some of them, such as secretory or mucinous, are usually low-grade and low stage tumors and have a good prognosis.
As indicated by Mutter and Prat in their Textbook (*Source:* Mutter GL, Prat J. Pathology of the Female Reproductive Tract, 3rd edition, Elsevier: UK), the diagnostic term "papillary" should be avoided as imprecise and potentially misleading. Papillary growth may be seen namely in both type-2 carcinomas, such as serous or clear cell, and type-1 carcinomas such as usual endometrioid carcinomas or several variants with mucinous, secretory or villoglandular differentiation.

Q.42 What is the best diagnostic designation for the endometrioid carcinoma shown in Figure 2.9?
  A. Villoglandular
  B. Secretory
  C. Mucinous
  D. Adenosquamous
  E. Papillary

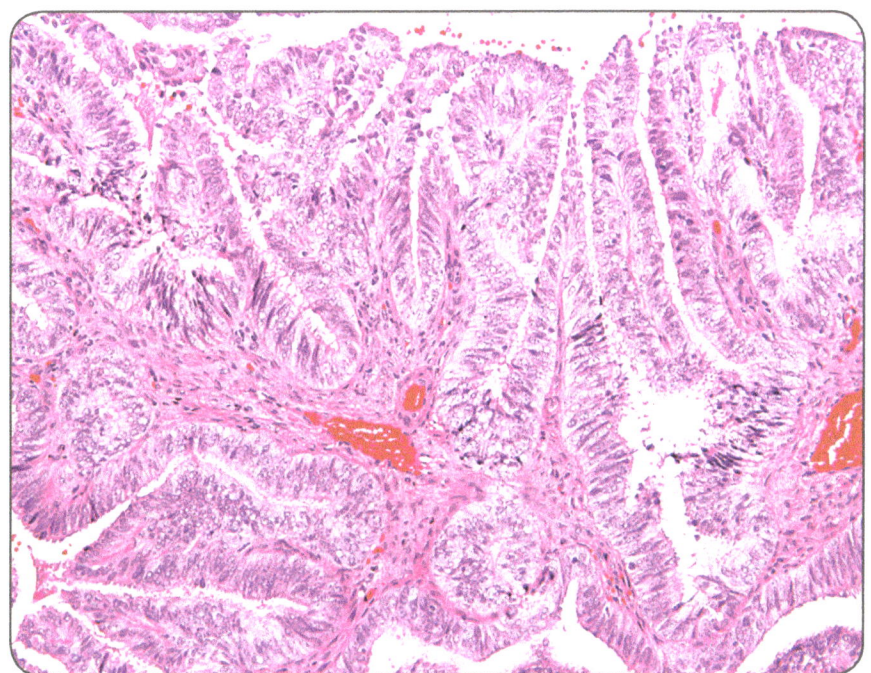

Figure 2.9

Answer: **A. Villoglandular**

Comment: The tumor cells line papillae with a fibrovascular core typical of the **villoglandular** growth pattern. Villoglandular structures are often seen admixed to other growth patterns and are typically most prominent in the luminal parts of the tumor.

Q.43 Which of the following is the most common histologic variant of endometrioid carcinoma of the uterus?
  A. Endometrioid adenocarcinoma with focal squamous differentiation
  B. Villoglandular endometrioid adenocarcinoma
  C. Secretory endometrioid adenocarcinoma
  D. Ciliated endometrioid adenocarcinoma
  E. Sertoliform endometrioid adenocarcinoma

Answer: **A. Endometrioid adenocarcinoma with focal squamous differentiation**

Comment: Classical **endometrioid adenocarcinoma with foci of squamous differentiation** account for approximately one-half of all endometrioid carcinomas. Villoglandular endometrioid adenocarcinoma account for one-third and all the other variants listed here as possible answers are less common.

Q.44 What is the best diagnosis for the endometrioid carcinoma shown in Figure 2.10?

A. Endometrioid adenocarcinoma with squamous differentiation
B. Villoglandular endometrioid adenocarcinoma
C. Secretory endometrioid adenocarcinoma
D. Ciliated endometrioid adenocarcinoma
E. Sertoliform endometrioid adenocarcinoma

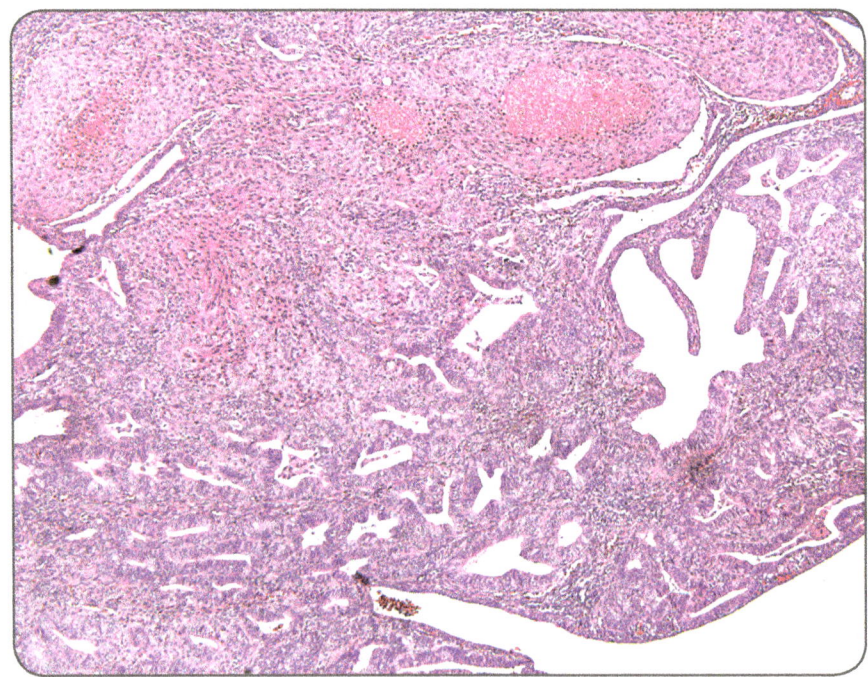

Figure 2.10

Answer: A. Endometrioid adenocarcinoma with squamous differentiation

Comment: The tumor consists of glands (lower part of the Figure 2.10) and nests of squamous epithelium occupying the entire upper part of the same figures. Some of the squamous nests show central necrosis. On the basis of these two elements the present tumor is best diagnosed as endometrioid **adenocarcinoma with squamous differentiation, grade 1.**

Q.45 Expressed in percentages, how many endometrioid carcinomas of the uterus occur in women under the age of 40 years?

A. 5%
B. 20%
C. 40%
D. 60%
E. 75%

Answer: A. 5%

Comment: Two-thirds of **endometrioid carcinoma** are found in **postmenopausal women**, and only 5% are diagnosed in women younger than 40 years of age. This may in part be due to the fact that small early tumors are often asymptomatic ("subclinical") and cause vaginal bleeding only after they have reached a certain critical size.

Q.46 An endometrioid adenocarcinoma in a hysterectomy specimen was found to be composed almost exclusively of glands, showing less than 5% of solid growth. The nuclei showed significant atypia with hyperchromatic clumped chromatin and prominent nucleoli. How should this tumor be classified using the criteria of the International Federation of Gynecology and Obstetrics (FIGO)?

- A. Grade I
- B. Grade II
- C. Grade III
- D. Grade I with a note of concern about the nuclear grade
- E. Grade II with a note that the tumor was upgraded due to nuclear atypia

Answer: E. Grade II with a note that the tumor was upgraded due to nuclear atypia

Comment: Tumors containing less than 5% of solid growth are signed out as grade I. However, if there is marked nuclear atypia, the tumors should be upgraded to grade II, with a note that this was done to account for nuclear atypia.

Q.47 What is the best diagnosis for the endometrial carcinoma shown in Figure 2.11?

- A. Endometrioid carcinoma, FIGO grade 1
- B. Endometrioid carcinoma, FIGO grade 2
- C. Endometrioid carcinoma, FIGO grade 3
- D. Secretory endometrioid carcinoma
- E. Sertoliform endometrioid carcinoma

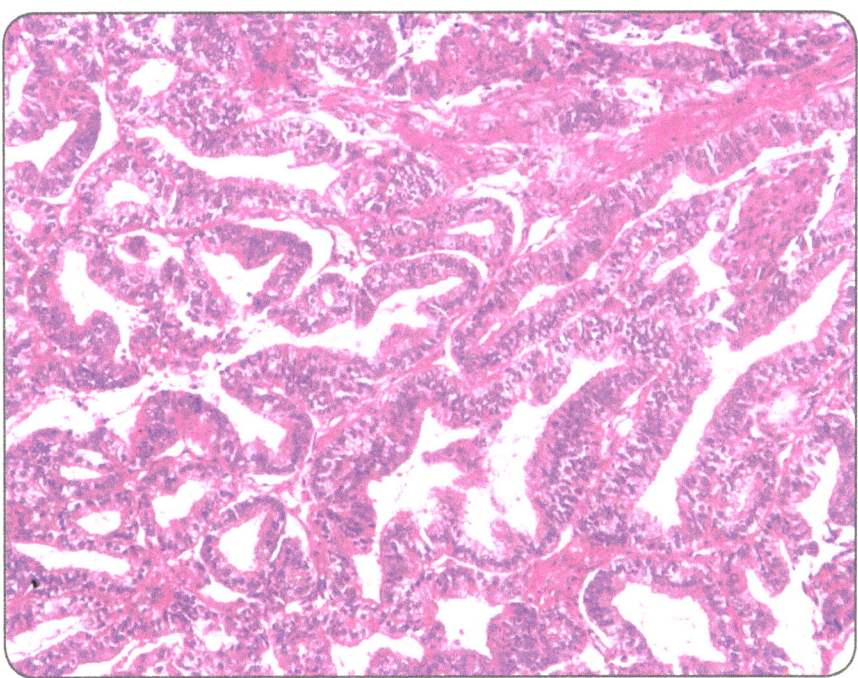

Figure 2.11

Answer: A. Endometrioid carcinoma, FIGO grade 1

Comment: The tumor is composed of endometrioid gland like structures, showing almost no solid growth, and it is thus designated as well-differentiated **endometrioid carcinoma, FIGO grade 1**.

Q.48 The gynecologist's decision to perform pelvic and para-aortic lymph node dissection is positively influenced by which of the following findings?

    A. Microinvasion of myometrium in 2–3 slides
    B. Microinvasion over a broad surface area of uterine cavity
    C. Depth of invasion of the myometrium of less than 50% of the myometrial wall thickness
    D. Invasion of the myometrium extending over 50% of the myometrial wall thickness
    E. Carcinoma extension into adenomyosis

Answer: D. Invasion of the myometrium extending over 50% of the myometrial wall thickness

Comment: Gynecologists base their decision on whether to perform pelvic and para-aortic lymph node dissection on three elements of the **pathology reports**:
- Extent and depth of invasion of myometrium
- Type of endometrial cancer (type-1 vs. type-2)
- Grade of the tumor.

Hysterectomy for tumors that have **penetrated through more than 50% of the thickness** of the myometrium is in most instance followed by lymph node dissection.

Microinvasion, which often difficult to assess, invasion of less than 50% of myometrial thickness and extension of carcinoma into adenomyosis are not indications for the dissection of pelvic and para-aortic lymph nodes, unless the tumor is high-grade.

Q.49 What is the best diagnosis for the endometrial carcinoma shown in Figure 2.12?

    A. Serous carcinoma
    B. Clear cell carcinoma
    C. Endometrioid adenocarcinoma
    D. Mucinous adenocarcinoma
    E. Undifferentiated carcinoma

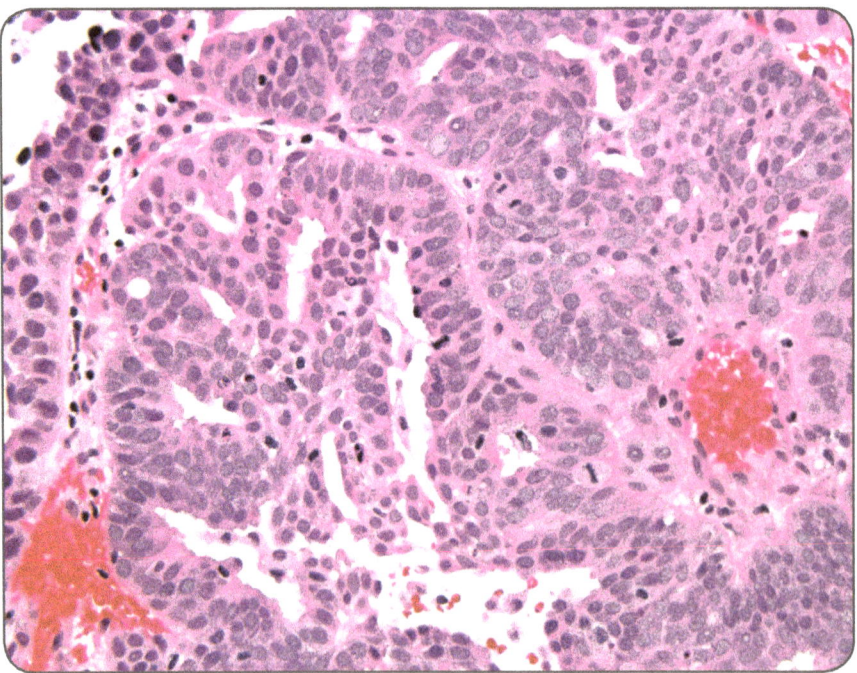

Figure 2.12

Answer: C. Endometrioid adenocarcinoma

Comment: This tumor is composed of glands lined by neoplastic cylindrical cells resembling proliferative endometrium, and solid areas exceeding 5% of the photographed field. Accordingly, this is an **endometrioid adenocarcinoma, FIGO grade 2.**

Q.50 An endometrial carcinoma was removed from a 70-year-old woman. The microscopic findings included broad-based papillae lined by high-grade cuboidal and pleomorphic cells. The cells had hyperchromatic nuclei with prominent nucleoli. They seemed to be overlapping one another and budding away from the papillae. These cells had scant amphophilic cytoplasm. Mitotic figures were prominent. There were a few scattered psammoma bodies. Tumor cells were also seen in the lymphatics of myometrium. What is the most likely diagnosis?

   A. Serous carcinoma
   B. Clear cell carcinoma
   C. Endometrioid carcinoma with secretory differentiation
   D. Endometrioid carcinoma, villoglandular variant
   E. Undifferentiated carcinoma

Answer: **A. Serous carcinoma**

Comment: This tumor resembles **high-grade serous carcinoma** of the ovary. Papillary growth with piling of the cells on the top of the papillae, with psammoma bodies, and lymphatic invasion of the myometrium are typical of these high-grade carcinomas type-2.

Q.51 What is the best diagnosis for this endometrial tumor removed from a 70-year-old woman (Figure 2.13)?

   A. Serous carcinoma
   B. Clear cell carcinoma
   C. Endometrioid carcinoma with secretory differentiation
   D. Endometrioid carcinoma, villoglandular variant
   E. Mucinous adenocarcinoma

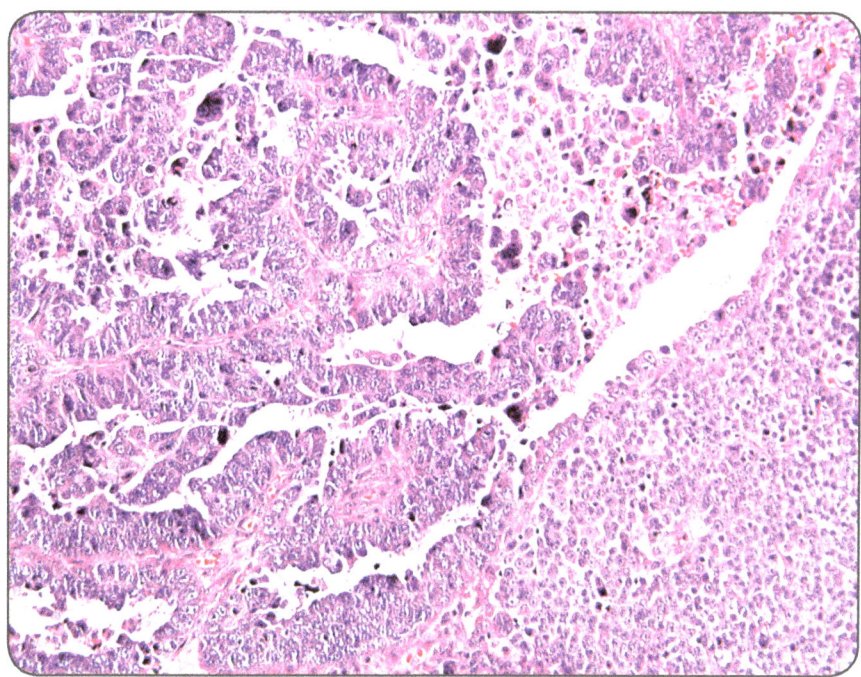

Figure 2.13

Answer: A. Serous carcinoma

Comment: The tumors shown in Figure 2.13 is composed of hyperchromatic cells lining irregular papillae on the left hand side and forming solid sheets on the right hand side of the figure. Thus, it represents a **serous carcinoma.**

Q.52 Which of the following microscopic findings is usually seen in the vicinity of invasive serous carcinoma of the endometrium?
- A. Endometrial hyperplasia without atypia
- B. Endometrial hyperplasia with atypia
- C. Serous endometrial intraepithelial carcinoma
- D. Endometrioid carcinoma
- E. Villoglandular endometrioid carcinoma

Answer: C. Serous endometrial intraepithelial carcinoma

Comment: **Serous endometrial intraepithelial carcinoma (EIC)** is found in the peritumoral endometrium in over 90% of cases of serous carcinoma. These malignant cells are not part of a precursor lesion, but a microscopic sign of intraepithelial spread of the serous carcinoma. Endometrial hyperplasia is not seen adjacent to these type II endometrial tumors, which typically do not results from unopposed estrogenic stimulation of the endometrium.

Q.53 What is the best diagnosis for this endometrial tumor removed from a 65-year-old woman (Figure 2.14)?
- A. Serous carcinoma
- B. Clear cell carcinoma
- C. Endometrioid carcinoma with secretory differentiation
- D. Endometrioid carcinoma, villoglandular variant
- E. Mixed adenocarcinoma

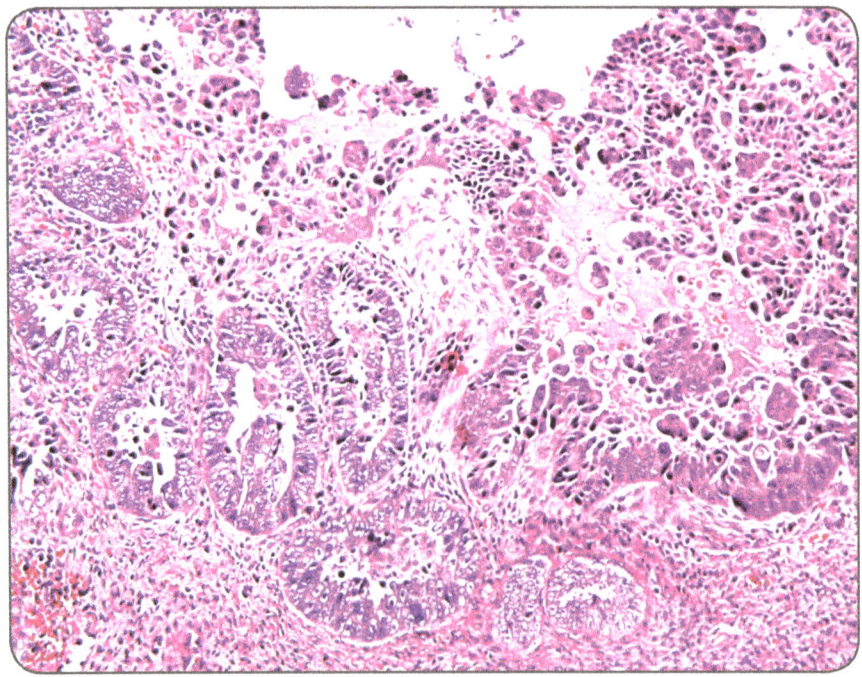

Figure 2.14

Answer: A. Serous carcinoma

Comment: The tumors shown in Figure 2.14 forms papillae on the right hand side of the figure and tubular glands lined by high-grade hyperchromatic cells of the same type and is thus best classified as papillary serous carcinoma. The tumor has no clear cell carcinoma or endometrioid features. This tumor should be distinguished from **mixed adenocarcinoma**, a tumor comprising high-grade papillary serous carcinoma and endometrioid carcinoma of low-grade (FIGO 1). It should be noted that one-third of all predominantly serous carcinomas of the endometrium contain high-grade endometrioid and clear cell carcinoma elements.

Q.54 Which of the following growth patterns may be seen in clear cell carcinoma of the endometrium?
  A. Hyalinized stroma enclosing tubular and cystic glands
  B. Papillary growth pattern
  C. Solid growth pattern
  D. Cystic growth pattern
  E. All of the above

Answer: E. All of the above

Comment: **Clear cell carcinoma** typically grows in several patterns, including **tubulocystic, papillary, and solid pattern**. Clear cells are best seen in solid areas. Glands and papillae may be lined by hobnailed cells. Stroma around the glands or in the core of the papillae is usually hyalinized.

Q.55 Carcinosarcomas of the internal female genital organs present most often in which form?
  A. As an endocervical mass
  B. As a bulky endometrial mass filling the uterine cavity
  C. As a myometrial nodule
  D. As a subserosal uterine mass
  E. As a solid ovarian mass

Answer: B. As a bulky endometrial mass filling the uterine cavity

Comment: **Carcinosarcomas** originate most often from the body of the uterus presenting as a bulky mass filling the uterine cavity. They are considered to be **metaplastic tumors** originating from the endometrium, sharing some genetic and epidemiological features with endometrioid carcinomas.

Q.56 Which form of sarcoma is most often seen in the sarcomatous component of uterine carcinosarcomas?
  A. Sarcoma, not otherwise specified (NOS)
  B. Leiomyosarcoma
  C. Liposarcoma
  D. Rhabdomyosarcoma
  E. Chondrosarcoma

Answer: A. Sarcoma, not otherwise specified (NOS)

Comment: The sarcomatous portion of **carcinosarcoma** is microscopically most often classified as NOS, resembling undifferentiated pleomorphic sarcoma of soft tissues. Some of these **homologous** sarcomas focally react with antibodies to smooth muscle cells or CD10 suggesting differentiation leiomyosarcoma or high grade endometrial stromal sarcoma. **Heterologous** differentiation into rhabdomyosarcoma, liposarcoma or chondrosarcoma is less common. Rhabdomyosarcoma is the most common of all the heterologous elements, but even if present it is seen only focally in the predominantly nondescript spindle cell sarcoma NOS. Microscopic identification of heterologous elements has no clinical significance.

Q.57 What is the best diagnosis for the endometrial tumor shown in Figure 2.15?

    A. Clear cell carcinoma
    B. Leiomyosarcoma
    C. Liposarcoma
    D. Rhabdomyosarcoma
    E. Carcinosarcoma

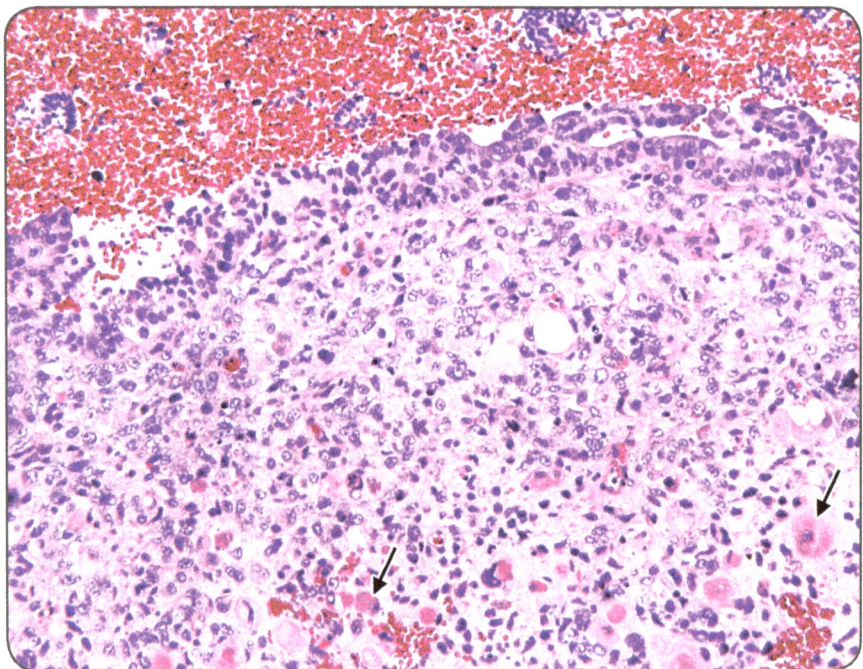

Figure 2.15

Answer: E. Carcinosarcoma

Comment: This carcinosarcoma has an adenocarcinoma component seen in the upper portion of the Figure 2.15, and a sarcoma component (the rest of the tumor). Apparently, the tumor is composed of malignant stromal cells. Focally, there is rhabdomyoblastic differentiation recognized by the eosinophilic cytoplasm of these cells (arrows).

Q.58 What is the best diagnosis for the endometrial tumor shown in Figure 2.16?

    A. Clear cell carcinoma
    B. Leiomyosarcoma
    C. Liposarcoma
    D. Carcinosarcoma, with homologous sarcoma component
    E. Carcinosarcoma, with heterologous sarcoma component

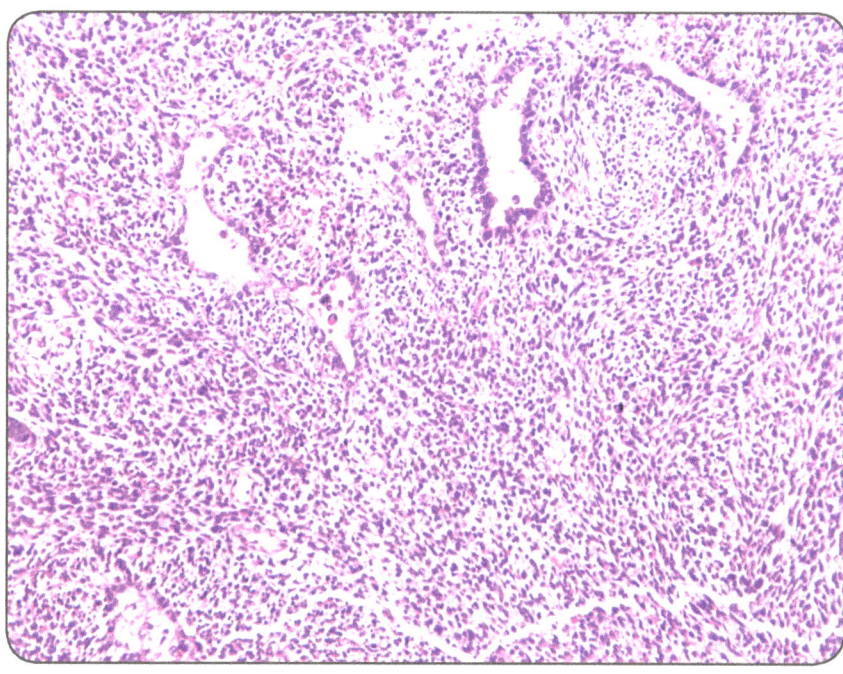

Figure 2.16

Answer: **D. Carcinosarcoma, with homologous sarcoma component**

Comment: This tumor contains an adenocarcinoma component (upper part) and a sarcoma component, which resembles endometrial stroma, i.e. an inherently **homologous** component of normal endometrium.

Q.59 What is the most likely diagnosis for the uterine tumor shown in Figure 2.17?

  A. Leiomyoma
  B. Leiomyosarcoma
  C. PEComa
  D. Endometrial stromal sarcoma, low-grade
  E. Endometrial stromal sarcoma, high-grade

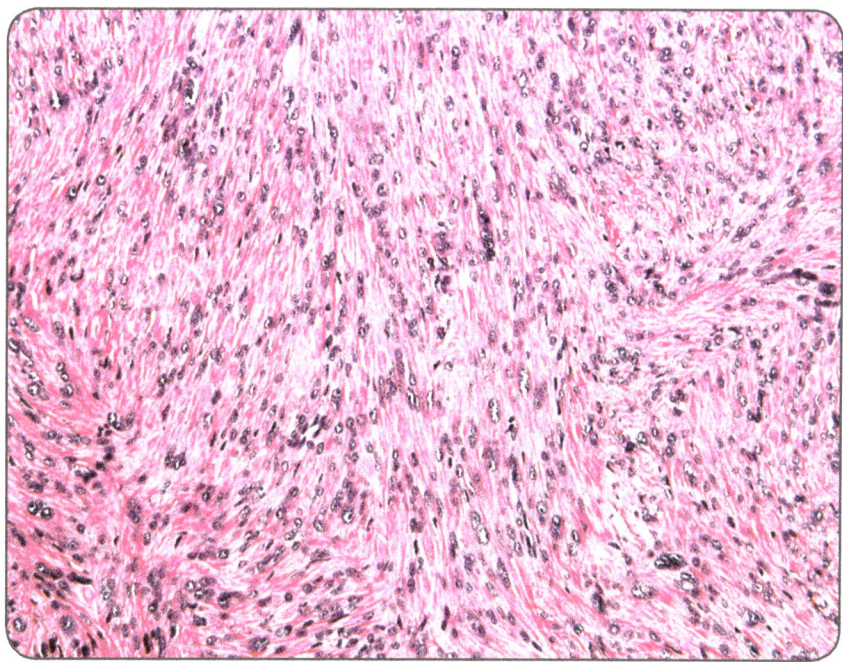

Figure 2.17

Answer: A. Leiomyoma

Comment: This tumor is composed of smooth muscle cells, i.e. cell with cigar-shaped nuclei and well-developed eosinophilic cytoplasm. The nuclei are relatively uniform, there are no mitotic figures and there is no necrosis, indicating that this is a benign tumor. On the basis of this observation one can exclude the diagnosis of leiomyosarcoma and high-grade endometrial stromal sarcoma. Tumor cells are not epithelioid and do not have a clear or granular cytoplasm to suggest the diagnosis of PEComa. Low-grade endometrial stromal sarcomas form tongue-like protrusions extending into the myometrium.

Q.60 A well-circumscribed 5 cm myometrial nodule, considered to be a leiomyoma on gross examination was found in a hysterectomy specimen of a 50-year-old woman diagnosed with uterine prolapse. Three sections of the nodule had the classical features of a leiomyoma, whereas the fourth slide showed the changes shown in Figure 2.18. There was no necrosis and mitoses were 2/per 10 high power fields. Immunohistochemistry revealed a low MIB-1 (Ki-67) count and the p53 was not expressed. What is the most likely diagnosis?

A. Highly cellular leiomyoma
B. Mitotically active leiomyoma
C. Apoplectic leiomyoma
D. Epithelioid leiomyoma
E. Leiomyoma with bizarre nuclei

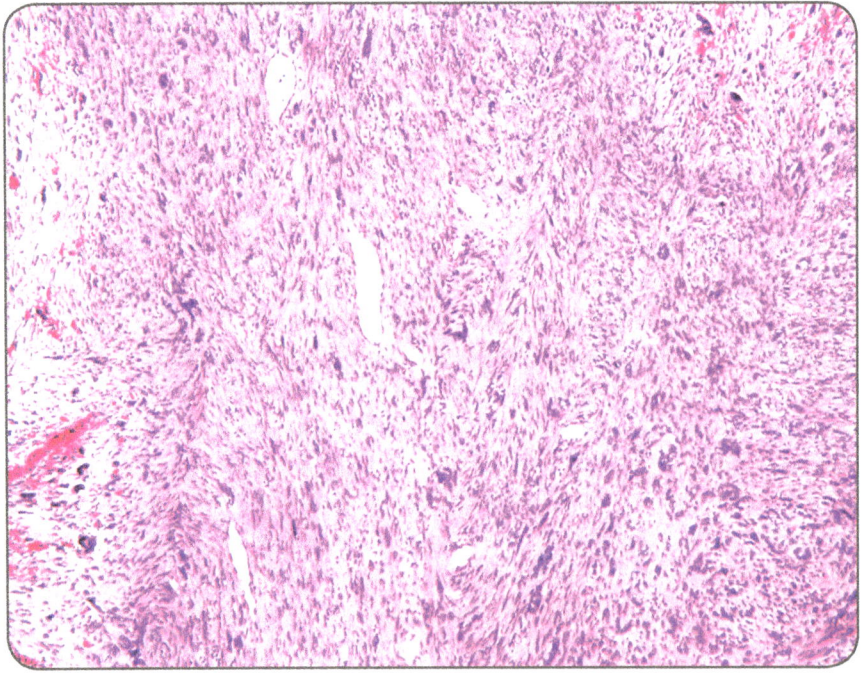

Figure 2.18

Answer: E. Leiomyoma with bizarre nuclei

Comment: Figure 2.18 shows a **leiomyoma with bizarre nuclei**, which appear hyperchromatic and have smudged chromatin. Immunohistochemistry also helps to distinguish this tumor from **leiomyosarcoma,** which usually shows areas of tumor necrosis, a high mitotic count, and a high MIB-1 count, as well as p53 expression. Focal appearance of these changes in an otherwise typical leiomyoma also supports the diagnosis; malignant transformation of leiomyoma is almost nonexistent.

Q.61 What is the most likely diagnosis of this 15 cm fleshy and partially necrotic myometrial tumor removed by hysterectomy from a 55-year-old woman (Figure 2.19)? The tumor was focal positive for desmin, and EMA and strongly positive for p53. MIB-1 count was high.

A. Leiomyosarcoma
B. Endometrial stromal sarcoma, low-grade
C. Perivascular epithelioid cell tumor
D. Lymphangioma
E. Gastrointestinal stromal tumor

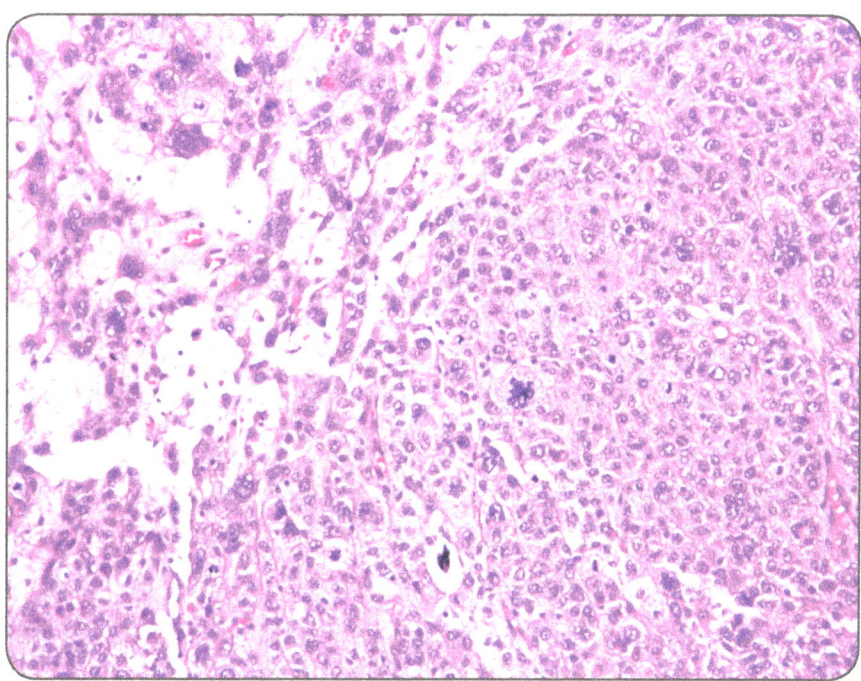

Figure 2.19

Answer: A. Leiomyosarcoma

Comment: This is an epithelioid **leiomyosarcoma** composed of lightly eosinophilic cells arranged in solid sheets. The term epithelioid leiomyosarcoma is used if more than 50% of cells have epithelioid features. Areas of necrosis were prominent but are not included in this microphotograph. Immunohistochemistry supported the diagnosis.

Q.62 A spindle cell well-circumscribed benign mesenchymal tumor was found in the myometrium. It was composed of tightly-packed cells with oval to round nuclei and clear cytoplasm arranged around thin-walled vessels. Tumor cells reacted with antibodies to smooth muscle cells and melanocytes (HMB45 and Melan A). What is the most likely diagnosis?

A. Leiomyoma
B. Endometrial stromal sarcoma
C. Perivascular epithelioid cell tumor
D. Lymphangioma
E. Gastrointestinal stromal tumor

Answer: C. Perivascular epithelioid cell tumor

Comment: **Perivascular epithelioid cell tumor (PEComa)** reacts with antibodies to smooth muscle cells and melanocytes. In contrast to leiomyomas which have eosinophilic cytoplasm and cigar-shaped elongated nuclei the nuclei of PEComas have oval to round nuclei and are in close contact with thin-walled blood vessels.

Q.63 Which of the following malignant tumors may occasionally present as a rare primary uterine malignancy?

A. Primitive neuroectodermal tumor (PNET)
B. Alveolar soft part sarcomas
C. Rhabdomyosarcoma
D. Yolk sac carcinomas
E. All of the above

Answer: E. All of the above

Comment: All the tumors listed here are occasionally found in the uterus, but are **extremely rare**. Some of them, like alveolar soft part sarcoma or rhabdomyosarcoma, occur more often in the cervix of young women than in the corpus of the uterus.

Q.64 Which part of the uterus is most often involved by primary lymphoma?

A. Cervix
B. Lower segment of endometrium
C. Fundus
D. Cornua
E. Myometrium

Answer: A. Cervix

Comment: Overall, **primary lymphoma of the female reproductive organs** is very rare. Such lymphomas usually involve the cervix or the ovaries, and are extremely uncommon in the corpus of the uterus (*Source:* Lemos S, et al. Eur J Gynecol Oncol. 2008; 29:656-8). On the other hand, **secondary** involvement of the uterus may be found in final stage of any disseminated lymphoma.

Q.65 A 3 cm well-circumscribed tumor was identified in the muscle wall of a hysterectomy specimen in a 40-year-old woman. It was composed of cells with uniform oval nuclei surrounded by eosinophilic cytoplasm. Tumor cells were arranged in anastomosing cords and trabeculae or forming vaguely outlined acini and tubules. No endometrial stromal sarcoma was identified. Tumor cells were positive for WT-1, smooth muscle cell actin, inhibin and CK7. What is the most likely diagnosis?

A. Granulosa cell tumor
B. PEComa
C. Endometrial stromal sarcoma, low-grade
D. Uterine tumor resembling sex cord stromal tumor
E. Adenomatoid tumor

Answer: D. Uterine tumor resembling sex cord stromal tumor

Comment: **Uterine tumor resembling sex cord stromal tumor (UTRSCT)** is a rare benign tumor composed of cells arranged in tubules and acini or forming cords and ribbons. Such tumors have a vague resemblance to **granulosa cell tumors** of the ovary. In contrast to ovarian granulosa cell tumors, they do not have the grooved nuclei and do not form Call-Exner like bodies. Tumor cells typically react with antibodies to smooth muscle cell actin or desmin, cytokeratin CK7 and WT-1, and less often antibodies to inhibin, calretinin and CD99. In a very small number of cases (less than 5%) tumors of this kind may recur, most likely because they contained coexistent **stromal endometrial sarcoma** (ESS) which was originally not identified. If ESS is identified, the tumor should be signed out as endometrial stromal sarcoma, low-grade, with extensive sex-cord like differentiation.

Other tumors listed here should be included in the differential diagnosis. **PEComas** are Melan A positive. **Adenomatoid tumors** are positive for mesothelioma markers such as CK 5/6, calretinin, or WT1.

Q.66 A submucosal polypoid 5 cm soft nodule protruding into the lumen of the uterus was found incidentally in a hysterectomy specimen in a 50-year-old woman. Microscopically, it was composed of small cell with round to oval nuclei and scant cytoplasm. Between the cells there were interspersed capillaries. These cells formed whorls around arterioles. There were no mitotic figures. Microscopically, the nodule was sharply demarcated from surrounding smooth muscle cells. The cells were positive for CD10, focally weakly positive for desmin and smooth muscle myosin, and negative for inhibin and Melan A. What is the most likely diagnosis?

   A. Endometrial stromal nodule
   B. Low-grade endometrial stromal sarcoma
   C. High-grade endometrial stromal sarcoma
   D. Undifferentiated endometrial stromal sarcoma
   E. Cellular leiomyoma

Answer: A. Endometrial stromal nodule

Comment: **Endometrial stromal nodule** is a benign lesion composed of cells resembling endometrial stromal cells arranged in a whorl-like pattern around arterioles. It differs from endometrial stromal sarcomas as it is not invading the lymphatics of the adjacent myometrium and does not show cytological signs of malignancy. Typically, it is CD10 positive and also weakly or focally positive for smooth muscle cell markers. Submucosal nodules are usually polypoid. Nodules found deeper in the myometrium may be mistaken for cellular leiomyoma. Leiomyomas react strongly with antibodies to smooth muscle cell markers, and are CD10 negative.

Q.67 A multinodular mass measuring 10 cm was identified in the wall of the uterus of an of a 50-year-old woman. It was distinct from normal myometrium, projecting into the uterine cavity. It was soft, yellow on cross-section and partially microcystic. Microscopically, it was composed of uniform blue spindle cells forming tongues which extended into the myometrium (Figure 2.20). There were 4 mitoses per 10 high power fields. Small foci of necrosis were often surrounded by foamy macrophages. Tumor cells were positive for CD10 and negative for smooth muscle cell markers. What is the most likely diagnosis?

   A. Endometrial stromal nodule
   B. Low-grade endometrial stromal sarcoma
   C. High-grade endometrial stromal sarcoma
   D. Undifferentiated endometrial stromal sarcoma
   E. Highly cellular leiomyoma

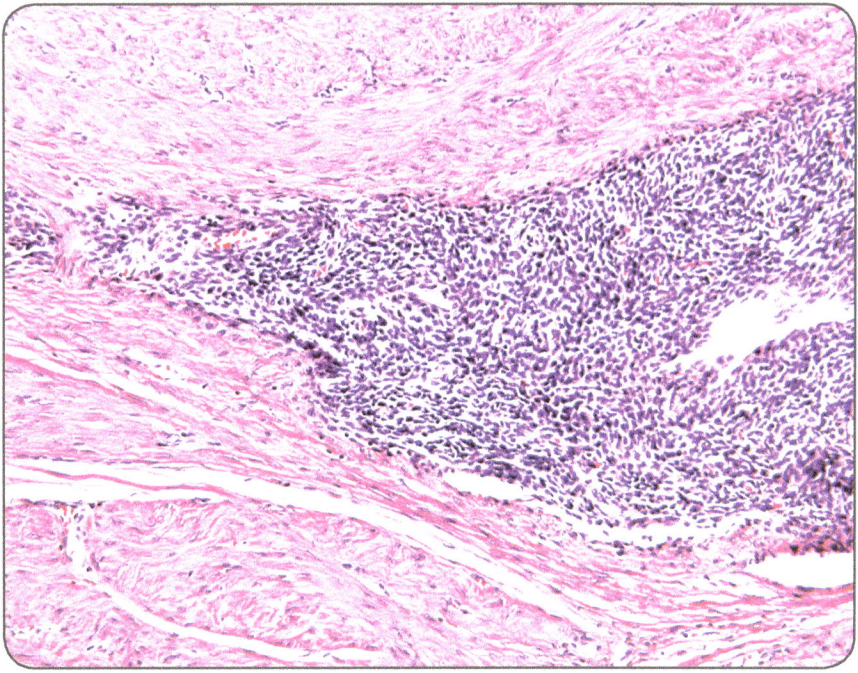

Figure 2.20

Answer: B. Low-grade endometrial stromal sarcoma

Comment: **Low-grade endometrial stromal sarcoma** is composed of cells that are identical to those seen in the endometrial stromal nodules. However, this tumor grows in an invasive manner forming typical tongue-like extensions in the adjacent myometrium and plugging the lymphatics. The presence of arterioles is yet another feature reminiscent of normal endometrial stroma. Areas of necrosis surrounded by foamy macrophages are common. Tumors are typically positive for CD10, but may show also smooth muscle cell differentiation, especially in the areas of hyalinization recognized by their characteristic "starburst pattern".

Q.68 Which microscopic forms of differentiation can be seen in low-grade endometrial stromal sarcomas?
- A. Smooth muscle
- B. Fibromyxoid
- C. Sex cord stromal-like
- D. Glandular
- E. All of the above

Answer: E. All of the above

Comment: **Low-grade endometrial stromal sarcomas** (ESS) may show numerous forms of **differentiation** which can be recognized microscopically or by immunohistochemistry. These additional microscopic features have no clinical or prognostic significance. However, for diagnostic purposes it is important to know that these forms of differentiation may occur in low-grade ESS.

Q.69 A 50-year-old woman had a hysterectomy for severe menorrhagia. A 3 cm grayish-white firm subserosal nodule was found in the fundus of the uterus which otherwise showed no other pathologic changes. Microscopically, it was composed of smooth muscle cells and tubular and cystic spaces lined by low cuboidal epithelium. These cells reacted with the antibodies to calretinin and cytokeratin CK5/6. What is the most likely diagnosis?
- A. Adenomyoma
- B. PEComa
- C. Endometrial stromal sarcoma, low-grade
- D. Uterine tumor resembling sex cord stromal tumor
- E. Adenomatoid tumor

Answer: E. Adenomatoid tumor

Comment: **Adenomatoid tumors** are benign tumors of mesothelial origin. Typically, they react with antibodies to mesothelial markers such as CK5/6 and calretinin. **Adenomyoma** is a rare benign smooth muscle cell tumor containing scattered endometrial glands surrounded by endometrial stroma. Most often they are intramural, but they may also be submucosal and subserosal. Other tumors listed here were discussed previously.

CHAPTER 3

Fallopian Tubes

Q.1 Fallopian tube is the most common site of extrauterine pregnancy. Which part of the fallopian tube most often contains the implantation site?

    A. Infundibular part
    B. Ampullary part
    C. Isthmus
    D. Interstitial part
    E. Intramural part

Answer: B. Ampullary part

Comment: The fallopian tube has four parts, which starting from the ovarian toward the uterine side include the following:
- Infundibulum
- Ampulla
- Isthmus
- Interstitial portion (also known as intramural part).
  Ectopic implantation most often occurs in the **ampullary part** of the fallopian tube. The implantation site can be recognized microscopically by the presence of extravillous (intermediate) trophoblast invading the tubal tissue.

Q.2 Which cells form the peritubal small cysts or small solid nests known as Walthard rests?

    A. Peritoneal cuboidal cells
    B. Squamous cells
    C. Transitional cells
    D. Ciliated cells
    E. Mucinous cells

Answer: C. Transitional cells

Comment: **Walthard rests** are made up of **transitional cells** with bland grooved nuclei. Cystic Walthard rests may contain proteinaceous eosinophilic material.

Q.3 What kind of metaplasia occurs most often in the fallopian tube of women who have been on chronic peritoneal dialysis?

    A. Transitional metaplasia
    B. Squamous metaplasia
    C. Mucinous metaplasia
    D. Endometrioid metaplasia
    E. Pseudocarcinomatous hyperplasia

Answer: B. Squamous metaplasia

Comment: **Squamous metaplasia** is a response to chronic irritation in dialysis patients. It may occur also in chronic salpingitis as part of the pelvic inflammatory disease.

Q.4 All the following diseases may cause or present in form of granulomatous salpingitis, *except:*
- A. Sarcoidosis
- B. Tuberculosis
- C. Actinomycosis
- D. Crohn disease
- E. Salpingitis isthmica nodosa

Answer: E. Salpingitis isthmica nodosa

Comment: **Salpingitis isthmica nodosa,** a common abnormality, analogous to adenomyosis of the uterus, is not a granulomatous disease.
Granulomatous salpingitis was previously a common feature of extrapulmonary or systemic miliary tuberculosis; however, today it is uncommon in the US and Europe. In typical cases, granulomas of tuberculosis show caseous necrosis. Other causes of infectious **granulomatous salpingitis**, such as *Actinomyces israeli* are also uncommon. Rare non-infectious causes of granulomatous salpingitis are Crohn disease and sarcoidosis. True granulomatous salpingitis must be distinguished from the more common **foreign body giant cell reaction** related to retained sutures or other surgical material.

Q.5 Bead-like nodularity was identified in the proximal part of the fallopian tube of a 45-year-old woman who underwent and hysterectomy for uterine leiomyomas together with bilateral salpingectomy. Microscopically, there were dilated gland-like structures between the smooth muscle fibers of the fallopian tubes. These gland-like spaces were lined by nonproliferative salpingeal epithelium. There was no acute or chronic inflammation. What is the best diagnosis?
- A. Follicular salpingitis
- B. Endosalpingiosis
- C. Endometriosis
- D. Salpingitis isthmica nodosa
- E. Xanthogranulomatous salpingitis

Answer: D. Salpingitis isthmica nodosa

Comment: **Salpingitis isthmica nodosa** (SIN) is a rather common finding in fallopian tubes removed for uterine or ovarian diseases. SIN may be identified upon careful microscopic examination in approximately 1% of all fallopian tubes, but even more often in surgically ligated tubes. The nodular part of the fallopian tube is composed of gland-like structures surrounded by fascicles of smooth muscles. It has been compared to uterine adenomyosis, except that the glands are not uterine but rather lined by fallopian tube-like epithelium.
Tubal endometriosis contains endometrial glands and endometrial stroma, which are not present in SIN.
Follicular salpingitis (a misnomer since it contains no follicles) is a chronic inflammation with fusion of the mucosal plicae imparting the cross-sectioned fallopian tube a complex glandular appearance with focal infiltrates of chronic inflammatory cells.
Endosalpingiosis refers to foci of fallopian tube-like epithelium in extratubal sites, such as lymph nodes. It may be found in the subserosal outer layer or muscle layer of fallopian tubes. In essence, it a form of "Müllerianosis" (ectopic Müllerian epithelium), or "endometriosis composed of tubal epithelium".
Xanthogranulomatous salpingitis is a form of chronic inflammation of fallopian tubes, which on gross examination appear deformed, swollen and yellow (*xanthos* in Greek means yellow). Microscopically, its chronic inflammatory infiltrate contains numerous foamy lipid laden macrophages, which account for the yellow color of the inflamed tissue.

Q.6 Which of the following is most likely to be found in women who have endometriosis?

　A. Follicular salpingitis
　B. Pseudoxanthomatous salpingitis
　C. Pseudocarcinomatous hyperplasia
　D. Granulomatous salpingitis
　E. Suppurative salpingitis

Answer: **B. Pseudoxanthomatous salpingitis**

Comment: **Pseudoxanthomatous salpingitis** with prominent foamy macrophages and hemosiderin deposits is a common finding in women who have **endometriosis** or had **tubal ligation**. In essence, it is a response to hemorrhage and accumulation of extravasated blood in tissues.

Q.7 What is the best diagnosis for this fallopian tube lesion (Figure 3.1)?

　A. Acute salpingitis
　B. Pseudoxanthomatous salpingitis
　C. Pseudocarcinomatous hyperplasia
　D. Granulomatous salpingitis
　E. Suppurative salpingitis

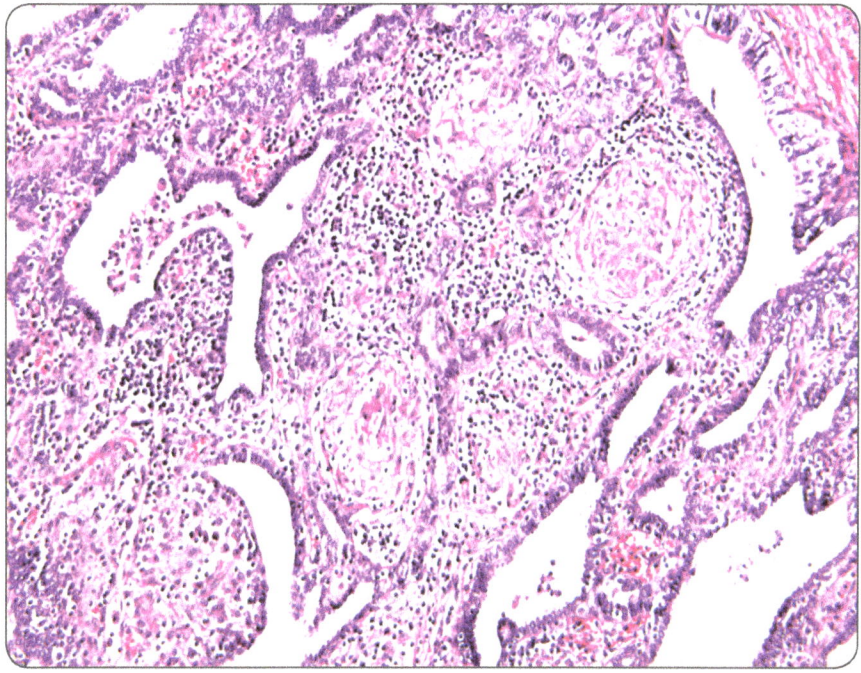

Figure 3.1

Answer: **D. Granulomatous salpingitis**

Comment: This microphotograph of fallopian tubes shows signs of chronic inflammation such as fusion of the plicae and foci of granulomatous inflammation. The patient had Crohn disease. To exclude tuberculosis all cases of granulomatous salpingitis should be stained with Ziehl-Neelsen stain for acid fast bacilli (AFB). We also include a Grocott methenamine silver stain to exclude fungi.

Q.8 Metaplastic papillary tumor (Figure 3.2) is typically found in which of the following groups of women?

A. Young nulliparous women
B. Pregnant women
C. Multiparous women of reproductive age
D. Perimenopausal women, 45 to 55 years of age
E. Older postmenopausal women, over 65 years of age

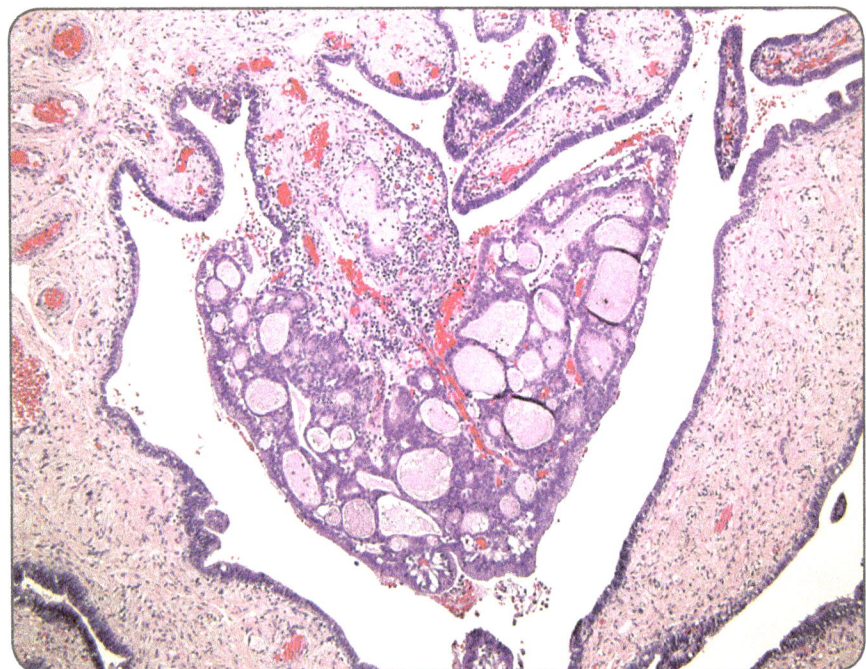

Figure 3.2

Answer: B. Pregnant women

Comment: **Metaplastic papillary tumor** is typically an incidental microscopic finding in **postpartum salpingectomy/tubal ligation specimens**. The lesion consists of papillae lined by metaplastic eosinophilic cuboidal to cylindrical epithelium. It is benign and should not be confused with preinvasive malignant tumors or their precursors.

Q.9 Several 1–3 mm red lesions were identified bilaterally on the subserosal part of the of the fallopian tubes of a 40-year-old woman (Figure 3.3). What is the most likely diagnosis?

A. Walthard nests
B. Mesothelial inclusion cysts
C. Endometriosis
D. Endosalpingiosis
E. Benign cystic mesothelioma

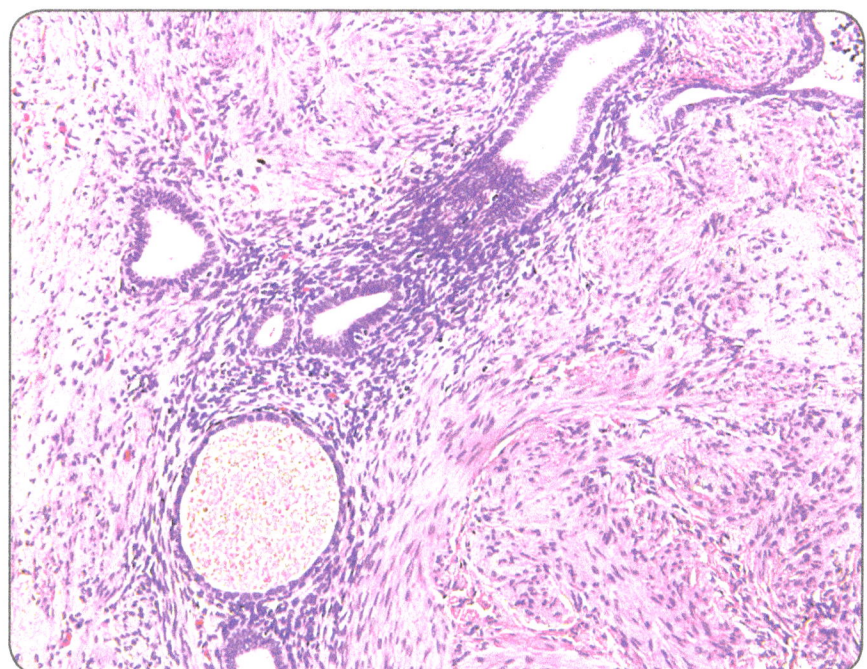

Figure 3.3

Answer: C. Endometriosis

Comment: The lesion consists of endometrial glands and stroma consistent with **endometriosis**. The dilated gland at 7 o'clock has even fragments pigmented material consistent with fragmented red blood cells from previous hemorrhage. Endosalpingiosis is similar to endometriosis but it contains no endometrial stroma and the glands are lined by ciliated tubal-like epithelium. Mesothelial inclusions and Walthard nests also lack endometrial stroma.

Q.10 This 2.5 cm nodule was identified in the wall of the fallopian tube of a 45-year-old woman (Figure 3.4). The tumor cells were positive for cytokeratin CK7 and calretinin. What is the most likely diagnosis?

A. Endometriosis
B. Salpingitis isthmica nodosa
C. Adenomatoid tumor
D. Lymphangioma
E. Malignant mesothelioma

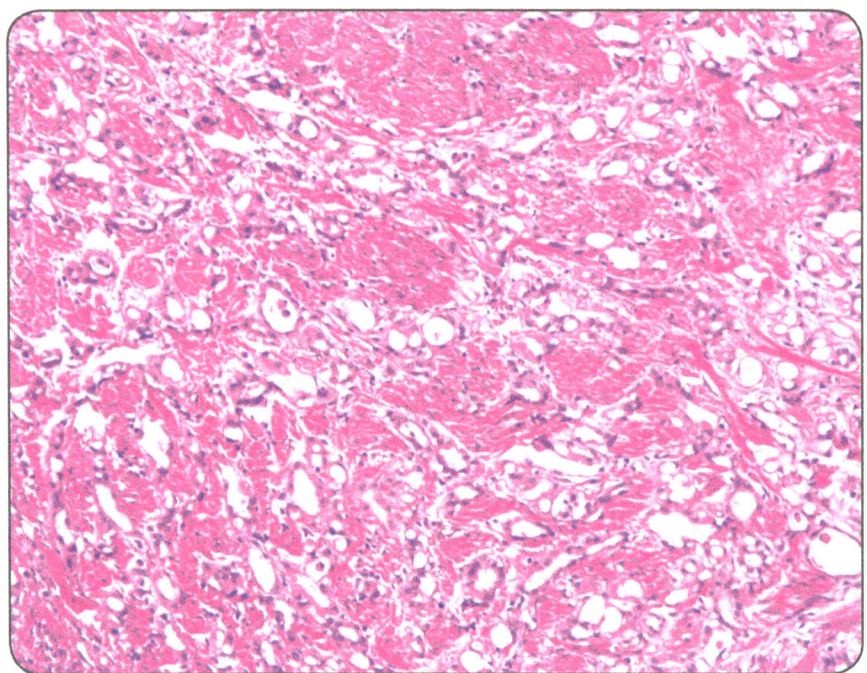

Figure 3.4

Answer: C. Adenomatoid tumor

Comment: **Adenomatoid tumor** is composed of tubular gland-like structures lined by flattened cuboidal epithelium, showing no signs of atypia, mitotic activity, apoptosis or necrosis. The tubular structures are surrounded by interlacing fibromuscular tissue. All other entities listed in this question deserve to be considered in the differential diagnosis.

Endometriosis comprises endometrial-like glands surrounded by typical endometrioid stroma, with signs of previous hemorrhage such as hemosiderin laden macrophages.

Salpingitis isthmica nodosa is composed of gland-like spaces lined by tubal epithelium. They are usually dilated and surrounded by fascicles of smooth muscle cells.

Lymphangioma may resemble adenomatoid tumors, but the dilated lymphatics are not lined by cytokeratin positive cells; like endothelial cells of the lymphatics, these cells express podoplanin and react with the antibody D2-40.

Malignant mesothelioma shows obvious macroscopic and microscopic signs of malignancy, and is usually much larger than the present tumor which measured only 1.5 cm in diameter. Malignant mesothelioma almost never presents as an isolated tubal lesion.

Q.11 All the following tubal lesions react with antibodies to p53, *except*:

A. Secretory cell outgrowths (SCOUT)
B. p53 signature lesion
C. Serous tubal intraepithelial neoplasia (STIN)
D. Serous tubal intraepithelial lesion (STIL)
E. Serous tubal intraepithelial carcinoma (STIC)

Answer: **A. Secretory cell outgrowths (SCOUT)**

Comment: Foci of secretory **cell outgrowths (SCOUT)**, also known as **benign epithelial hyperplasia,** are negative for p53. They consist of hyperplastic secretory cells, some of which may be ciliated, or endometrial-like epithelium showing pseudostratification.

p53 signatures are foci of tubal epithelium which by definition react with antibody to p53 but are composed of secretory cell showing only mild atypia.

Serous tubal intraepithelial neoplasia (STIN) is a low-grade p53 positive multilayered lesion which shows pseudostratification but only mild atypia and no loss of cellular polarity.

Serous tubal intraepithelial lesion (STIL) is a term used by some pathologists for the same lesions as STIN irrespective of the name to designate these lesions; none of them has the nuclear features of STIC.

Serous tubal intraepithelial carcinoma (STIC) is a readily recognizable intratubal malignancy, even though it does not show signs of invasion.

Expression of p53 in several tubal lesions shows that the diagnosis of such lesions should be based primarily on their microscopic morphology; immunohistochemistry for p53 has only an ancillary role, and should be used to confirm the microscopic diagnosis. It should be also noted that there are **p53 negative STICs**, which include a stop codon gene mutation not allowing the transcription of the p53 protein.

Q.12 All the following are typical features and essential for the diagnosis of serous tubal intraepithelial carcinoma (STIC), *except*:

A. Absence of ciliated cells
B. Multilayered arrangement of cells that have lost their polarity
C. Atypical cells with high nucleus-cytoplasm ratio
D. Horizontal fracture lines through the epithelium with dissociation of individual cells
E. Anisokaryosis

Answer: **E. Anisokaryosis**

Comment: **Serous tubal intraepithelial carcinoma (STIC)** is a lesion composed of secretory cells, which do not have cilia. The cells are arranged into several layers but have lost their polarity. Cells are obviously atypical and have a high nucleus-cytoplasm ratio. Cells tend to be discohesive and thus fracture lines form horizontally between the layers and some cells seem to dissociate from others. **Anisokaryosis**, i.e. variation in the size and shape of cells is relatively common in the fallopian tubes, and thus it is not an essential feature of STIC.

Q.13 Which of the following is the most common type of tubal carcinoma?

A. Serous carcinoma
B. Endometrioid carcinoma
C. Transitional cell carcinoma
D. Clear cell carcinoma
E. Squamous carcinoma

Answer: A. Serous carcinoma

Comment: More than 50% of all **primary tubal carcinomas** are **high-grade serous carcinomas**, which usually have solid areas. Transitional carcinomas are also classified as serous. It is worth notice that many of these tumors present by their dominant ovarian extension, and therefore, the primary site cannot be always determined. The presence of STIC adjacent to the invasive carcinoma in such cases is taken as the best evidence that the tumor is of tubal origin.

Q.14 What is the best diagnosis for the tubal carcinoma shown in Figure 3.5?
   A. High-grade serous carcinoma
   B. Endometrioid carcinoma
   C. Transitional cell carcinoma
   D. Clear cell carcinoma
   E. Squamous carcinoma

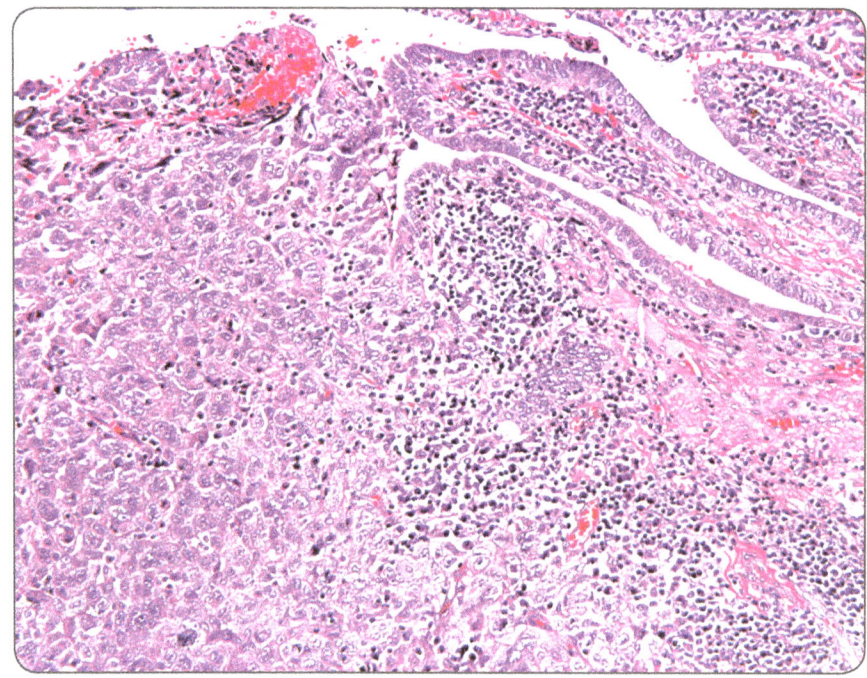

Figure 3.5

Answer: A. High-grade serous carcinoma

Comment: This tumor is composed of hyperchromatic cuboidal cells lining the fimbriae of the fallopian tube mucosa in continuity with an almost solid neoplastic mass occupying most of the field, which is typical of **high-grade serous carcinoma**.

Q.15 A 6 cm solid tumor was found on the outer subserosal portion of the fallopian tube of a 53-year-old woman. The tumor was composed of relatively bland cells forming tubules, solid sheets and small cysts. Tumor cells had scant cytoplasm and their nuclei were oval, pale, and had no grooves. The tumor was positive for cytokeratin CK7 and CAM5.2, CD10, calretinin and focally for inhibin. It was negative for EMA and CEA. It was also negative for cytokeratin CK5/6, podoplanin (D2-40), and WT1. What is the most likely diagnosis?

A. Low-grade serous carcinoma
B. Granulosa cell tumor
C. Female adnexal tumor of Wolffian origin (FATWO)
D. Adenomatoid tumor
E. Malignant mesothelioma

Answer: C. Female adnexal tumor of Wolffian origin (FATWO)

Comment: **Female adnexal tumor of Wolffian origin (FATWO)** is a benign tumor thought to originate from mesonephric (Wolffian) remnants on the surface of fallopian tubes, mesosalpinx or mesoovary. With a few rare exceptions, most reported cases had good prognosis.

FATWO is composed of bland cells forming cords, sheets, as well as tubules and cysts in a sieve-like manners. By immunohistochemistry it is positive for cytokeratin CK7 (CAM5.2) and CK19, CD10, vimentin and calretinin. It is focally positive for inhibin and consistently negative for EMA. It does not have grooved nuclei, like those seen in **granulosa cell tumors**. It forms tubules like **adenomatoid tumor**, but in contrast to that tumor of peritoneal origin, it does not react with antibodies to cytokeratin CK5/6, D2-40 and WT1. **Endometrioid carcinoma** metastatic to the fallopian tube must be excluded as well.

CHAPTER 4

Ovary

Q.1 Which cells form the Call-Exner bodies in the normal ovary?

A. Oocytes
B. Granulosa cells
C. Theca interna cells
D. Theca externa cells
E. Cortical stromal cells

Answer: B. Granulosa cells

Comment: Call-Exner bodies are formed by **granulosa cells** which aggregate around a centrally positioned acellular eosinophilic spherule composed of extracellular matrix and secretory material. Similar bodies are formed by the neoplastic granulosa cells. These bodies were first described in the rabbit ovary by Emma Louise Call and Sigmund Exner (1875), and deservedly carry their name.

Q.2 Figure 4.1 shows the perihilar tissue of a normal ovary of a postmenopausal woman. The polygonal cells with eosinophilic cytoplasm shown here in the vicinity of nerves and small blood vessels react with the antibody to which of the following antigens?

A. Cytokeratin 20
B. Chromogranin
C. Inhibin
D. Secretin
E. Prolactin

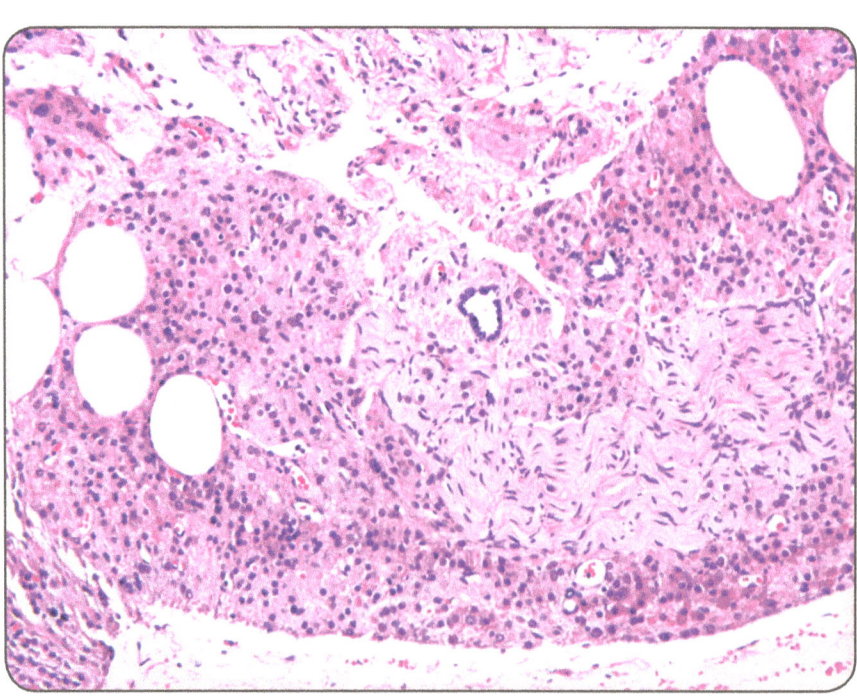

Figure 4.1

Answer: **C. Inhibin**

Comment: Figure 4.1 shows aggregates of **hilar cells** in the mesovarium, commonly found in postmenopausal women. These cells have eosinophilic cytoplasm, which typically reacts with antibodies to **inhibin**. There are two types of inhibin (inhibin A and inhibin B), but most pathology laboratories use antibodies to inhibin A. Hilar cells resemble testicular Leydig cells and may contain Reinke crystals. They are also calretinin positive. Similar groups of cells may be seen inside the ovary itself, usually in the hilum.

Q.3 What is the best diagnosis for the ovarian cyst shown in Figure 4.2?

    A. Unluteinized follicular cyst
    B. Granulosa lutein cyst
    C. Theca lutein cyst
    D. Corpus luteum cyst
    E. Corpus albicans cyst

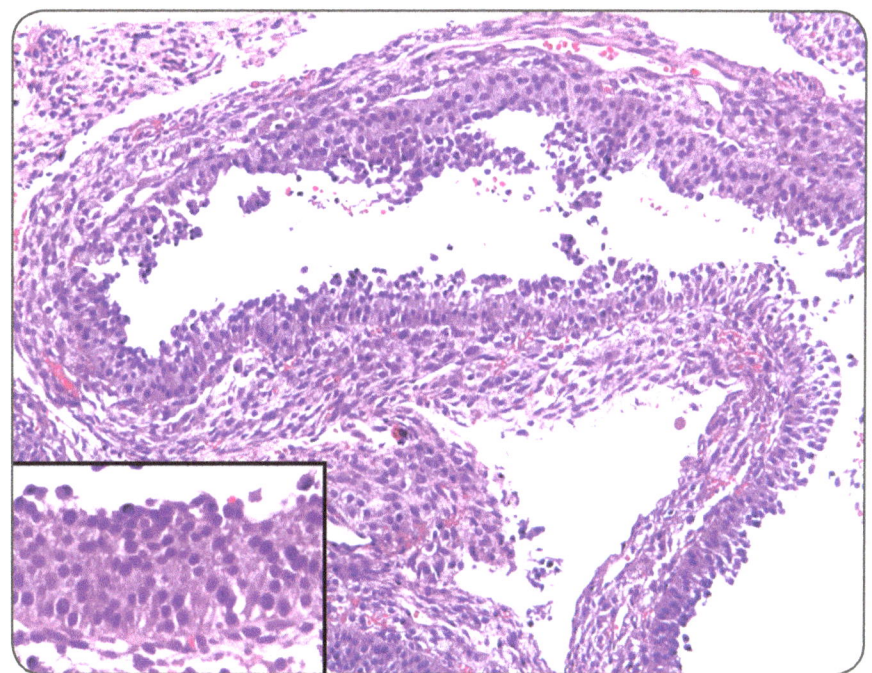

Figure 4.2

Answer: **B. Granulosa lutein cyst**

Comment: This cyst shown in Figure 4.2 is lined by luteinized granulosa cells. These cells are cuboidal and have eosinophilic cytoplasm.

Q.4 Which ovarian cysts predominantly produce estrogens?

    A. Unluteinized follicular cysts
    B. Theca lutein cysts
    C. Granulosa lutein cysts
    D. Corpus luteum cysts
    E. Corpus albicans cysts

Answer: A. Unluteinized follicular cysts

Comment: **Unluteinized follicular cysts** are lined by granulosa cells which predominantly secrete estradiol.

Theca lutein cysts secrete androstenedione.

Granulosa lutein cysts are lined by luteinized granulosa cells, which secrete progesterone. In this respect, granulosa lutein cysts resemble **corpus luteum cysts.**

Clinically, all these cysts are classified as **functional cysts**, in contrast to **nonfunctional cysts** which include **corpus albicans cysts** and those related to **endometriosis** or **mesothelial inclusion cysts** and cystadenomas.

Q.5 Which of the following statements is true of luteoma of pregnancy (Figure 4.3)?
- A. They usually present clinically during the first trimester of pregnancy
- B. Approximately 80% of luteomas of pregnancy occur in African-American women
- C. They are usually cystic
- D. They are almost always unilateral
- E. Cells of these lesions contain abundant lipid droplets

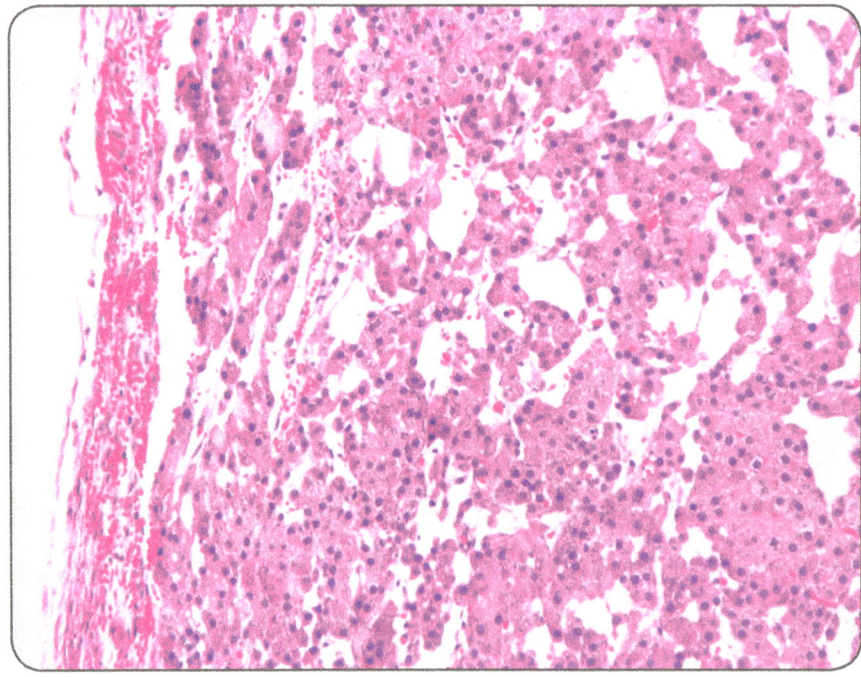

Figure 4.3

Answer: B. Approximately 80% of luteomas of pregnancy occur in African-American women

Comment: For unknown reasons **luteomas of pregnancy** show marked racial predominance and are in approximately 80% of cases found in African-American women. They are diagnosed usually in the third trimester of pregnancy. They present as solid nodules or solid masses, which are usually found in both ovaries. Microscopically, they are composed of cuboidal cells that have have small round nuclei and well-developed eosinophilic cytoplasm (Figure 4.3). In contrast to steroid cell tumors of the ovary, which microscopically may resemble these pregnancy lesions, luteoma cells contain no or only minimal amounts of lipid.

Q.6 Which of the following diseases is most often associated with hyperreactio luteinalis presenting in pregnancy in form of bilateral multiple theca lutein cysts?

A. Diabetes mellitus
B. Preeclampsia
C. Hyperemesis gravidarum
D. Hydatidiform mole
E. Placenta accreta

Answer: **D. Hydatidiform mole**

Comment: **Bilateral theca lutein cysts ("hyperreactio luteinalis")** are found in 25% of **molar pregnancies**, as well as those associated with choriocarcinoma. Elevated levels of serum hCG play an important role in the pathogenesis of these cysts, although it is obvious that other conditions must be present for the cysts to arise. Other conditions that may be associated with bilateral theca lutein cysts include the following:
- Multiple fetuses
- Immune hydrops fetus
- Non-immune hydrops fetus
- Maternal chronic renal failure

Bilateral theca lutein cysts involute spontaneously during the postpartum period. Sometimes they may cause multicystic enlargement of the ovaries during pregnancy and may be mistaken during cesarean section or other surgical procedures for cystic tumors.

Q.7 In polycystic ovary syndrome, which of the following parts of the ovary becomes widened and more densely collagenous than in a normal ovary?

A. Outer fibrous part of the cortex
B. Inner cellular part of the cortex
C. Layer of the cortex that contains oocytes
D. Medulla
E. Hilum

Answer: **A. Outer fibrous part of the cortex**

Comment: In **polycystic ovary syndrome** (PCOS), which is characterized by hyperandrogenism and oligo-ovulation or anovulation, the ovary shows typical but otherwise non-diagnostic changes. These include collagenous widening of the **outer fibrous part of the cortex** and numerous **cystic antral follicles** in the inner part of the cortex (i.e. the part which normally contains the oocytes). The outer cortical layer, which is normally fibrotic and acellular, becomes wider and more collagenous resembling an **"ovarian capsule"**. The cystic follicles are typically uniform and show theca cell hyperplasia, reflecting the common excessive LH stimulation of the ovaries. None of these ovarian changes is diagnostic of PCOS, and all of them may be found in other anovulatory conditions. The medulla and hilum are not altered in PCOS.

Q.8 A 25-year-old woman with a history of menstrual irregularities, infertility and mild masculinization presented with lower abdominal pain on the left side. A palpable solid left adnexal mass measuring 15 cm was identified by ultrasound. The contralateral ovary appeared normal. An intraoperative wedge biopsy revealed edema of the medulla and sparing of the cortex, which appeared normal (Figure 4.4). No carcinoma or lymphoma cells were identified by immunohistochemistry. What is the most likely diagnosis?

A. Torsion of the ovary
B. Massive ovarian edema
C. Fibroma of the ovary
D. Sclerosing stromal tumor of the ovary
E. Krukenberg tumor

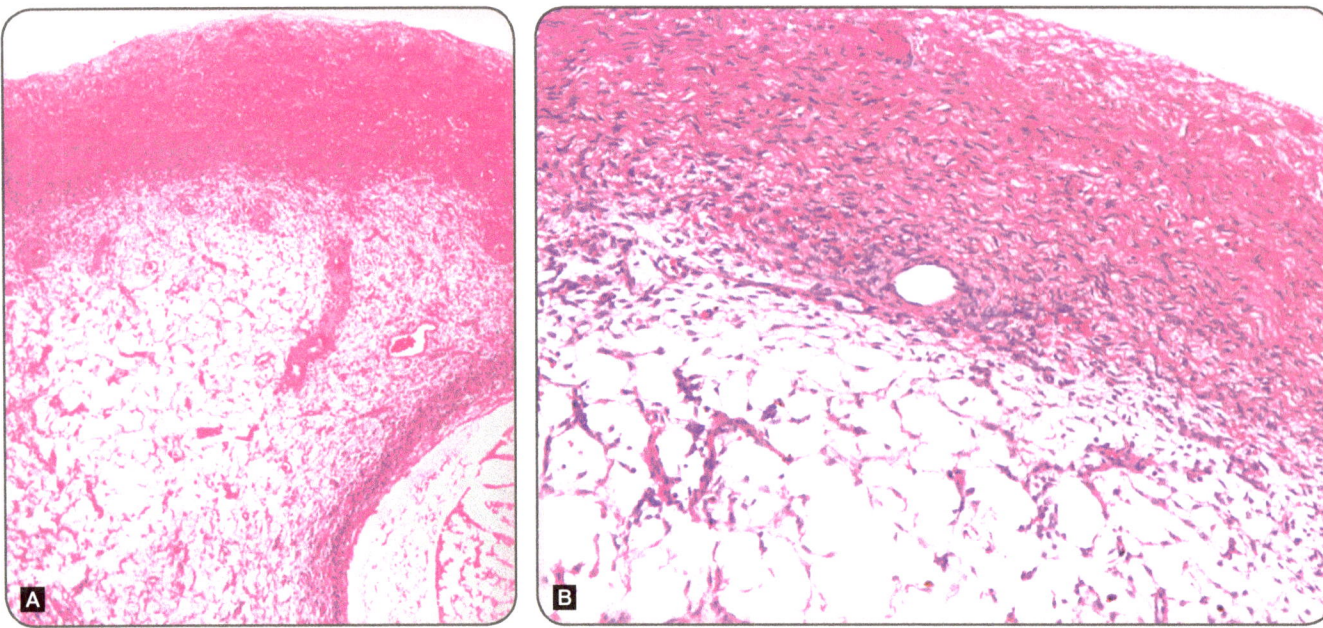

Figures 4.4A and B

Answer: B. Massive ovarian edema

Comment: Edema of the medulla and sparing of the cortex (Figure 4.4A and B), with no evidence of neoplasia on frozen section as well as by immunohistochemistry, is most consistent with the diagnosis of **massive ovarian edema**. The cause of this rare ovarian disease is not known. It has been hypothesized that edema results from partial or recurrent ovarian torsion, even though there is no histological evidence of necrosis or ischemia. As in the present case, the condition may be associated with hormonal changes, even those suggesting PCOS.

All the tumors listed as alternative answers need to be excluded on wedge biopsy, especially if one is contemplating preservation of the ovary.

Fibromas and **sclerosing stromal tumor** of the ovary may be edematous, but in those cases edema involves only the tumor and not the ovary itself. Fibroma is however a tumor of older women, with a peak incidence between 50 and 60 years of age; it is unlikely that it would develop in a 25-year-old woman. Sclerosing stromal tumors occur in the 25-year age group but these tumors have a pseudolobular appearance and tend to compress the ovary.

Krukenberg tumor may cause massive edema, but it is usually bilateral and it is usually found in women who are older than the present patient. In the third decade, one should also consider ovarian **lymphoma**, which may be quite edematous.

In women under the age of 30 years the differential diagnosis should include ovarian fibromatosis, a condition not mentioned in this question. **Fibromatosis of the ovary** is a non-neoplastic condition closely-related to massive ovarian edema, that also may cause enlargement of the ovary. The ovary is lobulated on cross-section and firm. Microscopically, there is dense collagenous matrix enclosing spindle cells that are arranged in a storiform or fascicular manner. Spindle cells extend between the relatively well-preserved normal elements involving the cortex as well as the medulla.

The pathologic entities to be included in the differential diagnosis of massive ovarian edema are included in the Table 4.1.

Table 4.1: Differential diagnosis of massive ovarian edema

Non-neoplastic conditions	• Fibromatosis of the ovary
Benign tumors	• Fibroma • Fibrothecoma • Sclerosing stromal tumor of the ovary
Malignant tumors	• Metastatic adenocarcinoma of GI origin (Krukenberg tumor) • Metastatic goblet cell carcinoid of GI origin • Lymphoma of the ovary

Ovary

Q.9 Pathologic examination of the ovaries and tubes removed for clinically diagnosed adnexal/ovarian torsion in children will not reveal an underlying pathologic cause of the torsion in how many instances, as expressed in percentages?

   A. Less than 2% (i.e. the cause will be found in essentially all cases)
   B. Less then 10%
   C. Approximately 30%
   D. Approximately 50%
   E. More than 85%

Answer: C. Approximately 30%

Comment: **Ovarian torsion** almost always involves a torsion of the fallopian tube and therefore it is more appropriate to call it **tubo-ovarian** or **adnexal torsion**. Torsion can occur at any age, including the neonatal period, childhood, and very old age. No identifiable pathologic cause for the torsion could be found in approximately **30% of children** clinically diagnosed to have adnexal torsion. In contrast to children, **adnexal torsion in adults** is most often caused by pathologic processes that cause enlargement of the ovaries. Hence, tumors are a common cause of adnexal torsion in adult women. An increased incidence of adnexal torsion also has been recorded in the first trimester of pregnancy, most likely due to increased mobility of the adnexa in early pregnancy.

Q.10 What is the most common cause of an afollicular premature ovarian failure ("premature follicular depletion")?

   A. Unknown (idiopathic)
   B. Autoimmune
   C. Iatrogenic
   D. Environmental
   E. Genetic

Answer: A. Unknown (idiopathic)

Comment: The cause of premature follicular depletion resulting in premature ovarian failure cannot be identified in most instances, and it is thus considered to be **idiopathic.** Identifiable causes listed in this question are less common.

Q.11 All the following are constant clinical features of premature ovarian failure, *except:*

   A. Amenorrhea for 4–6 months
   B. Age under 40 years
   C. High serum FSH exceeding 30 IU/L
   D. Hypoestrinism
   E. Evidence of virilization

Answer: E. Evidence of virilization

Comment: **Premature ovarian failure** (POF) is defined as amenorrhea of 4–6 months duration beginning under the age of 40 years, and associated with postmenopausal levels of FSH (>30 IU/L) and hypoestrinism. Virillization may be present but it is not a constant feature of POF.

Q.12 An infertile 30-year-old woman with typical signs of autoimmunity involving several organs had an ovarian wedge biopsy, which is shown in this Figure 4.5. Which autoantibodies are most likely to be found in this woman?

   A. Anti-adrenal antibodies
   B. Anti-thyroid antibodies
   C. Anti-islet cell antibodies
   D. Anti-parathyroid antibodies
   E. Anti-pituitary antibodies

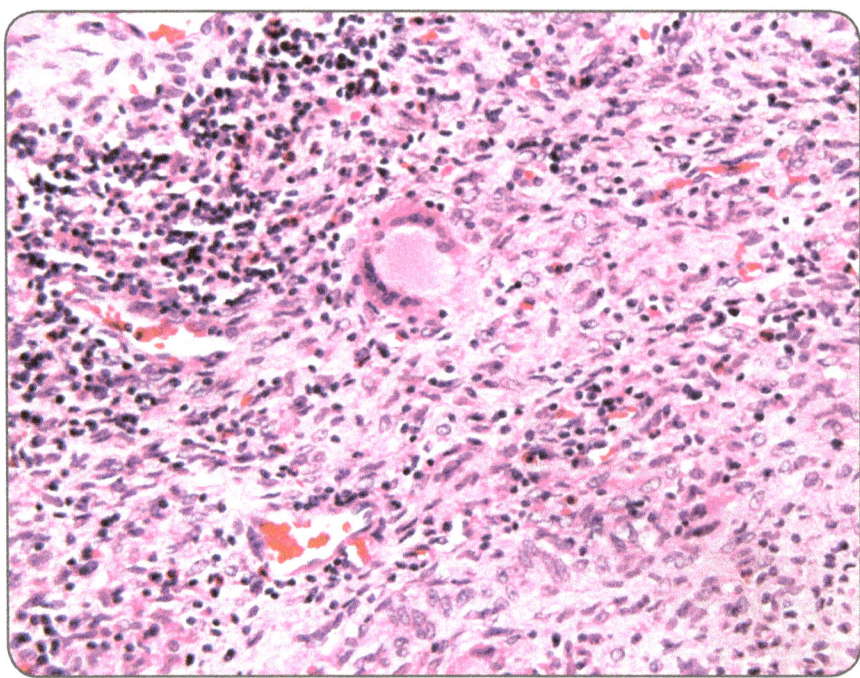

Figure 4.5

Answer: A. Anti-adrenal antibodies

Comment: Microscopic signs of **autoimmune oophoritis**, marked by infiltrates of lymphocytes, plasma cells and macrophages and multinucleated giant cells (Figure 4.5) are usually associated with signs of autoimmune adrenalitis and anti-adrenal antibodies in serum. Many other antibodies may be found in women with autoimmune infertility, but these serologic signs of autoimmune diseases usually do not cause autoimmune oophoritis.

Q.13 Severe ovarian hyperstimulation syndrome (OHSS) induced by clomiphen is characterized by ovarian enlargement. What is the predominant microscopic finding in such ovaries?

  A. Multiple corpora lutea cysts
  B. Multiple non-luteinized follicular cysts
  C. Multiple granulosa-lutein cysts
  D. Multiple theca-lutein cysts and one or more corpora lutea
  E. Cortical stromal hyperplasia

Answer: D. Multiple theca-lutein cysts and one or more corpora lutea

Comment: **Ovarian hyperstimulation syndrome** (OHSS) is classified as mild, moderate or severe. In the **severe form of OHSS,** there are numerous theca-lutein cysts and one or several corpora lutea.

Q.14 Acute vascular changes induced by radiation of the ovary and mesovarium are most prominent in which blood vessels?

  A. Arteries
  B. Arterioles
  C. Capillaries
  D. Venules
  E. Veins

Answer: **A. Arteries**

Comment: Microscopic **vascular changes induced by radiation** of ovaries and mesovarium are most prominent in arteries, although it is believed that most of the tissue damage induced by radiation is caused by the damage of small blood vessels. The most common microscopic changes include fibrinoid necrosis of the arterial wall, thrombi, foam cell accumulation in the intima, and myointimal proliferation of fibroblasts and myofibroblasts.

Q.15 What is the most likely cause of massive hemorrhage from the right ovary?
- A. Follicular cyst
- B. Corpus luteum
- C. Corpus albicans
- D. Endometriosis
- E. Massive edema of the ovary

Answer: **B. Corpus luteum**

Comment: **Ruptured corpora lutea** are the most common cause of profuse ovarian hemorrhage. Such hemorrhage is uncommon, but 65% of massive bleedings occur from the **right ovary,** usually between day 21 and 26 of the normal 28 day menstrual cycle. The reasons for the bleeding are not known, neither it is known why the **right ovary** is involved more often than the left ovary. Pregnancy and congenital or acquired coagulopathies increase the risk of massive ovarian hemorrhage. Pathologic examination of the wedge biopsy of the ovary will usually identify a partially necrotic corpus luteum as the most likely cause of the bleeding. Luteinized cells, shed from the ruptured corpus luteum, may be seen in the clotted blood removed from the peritoneal cavity.

Q.16 Which of the following is the most common malignant ovarian tumor accounting for approximately 70% of all primary ovarian carcinomas?
- A. High-grade serous carcinoma
- B. Endometrioid carcinoma
- C. Clear cell carcinoma
- D. Mucinous carcinoma
- E. Low-grade serous adenocarcinoma

Answer: **A. High-grade serous carcinoma**

Comment: **High-grade serous carcinoma** (HGSC) is the most common malignant ovarian tumor accounting for approximately 70% of all carcinomas, which in turn represent over 95% of all ovarian malignant tumors.

Q.17 Expressed in percentages, how many serous ovarian tumors are benign?
- A. 10%
- B. 25%
- C. 50%
- D. 70%
- E. >90%

Answer: **D. 70%**

Comment: Approximately, 70% of all **serous ovarian tumors** are benign, up to 10% are borderline and 20–25% are carcinomas.

Q.18 Expressed in percentages, how many serous borderline tumors (SBT) are bilateral at the time of diagnosis?

A. Less than 10%
B. Approximately 33%
C. Approximately 50%
D. Approximately 66%
E. More than 90%

Answer: B. Approximately 33%

Comment: Approximately, 33% (one-third) of all **serous borderline tumors** are bilateral at the time of diagnosis. In contrast to these tumors, only 20% serous cystadenomas are bilateral. Approximately, 60% of high-grade serous carcinomas are bilateral.

Q.19 Expressed in percentages, how many serous borderline tumors have spread beyond the ovaries and involve the pelvis or abdominal organs at the time of diagnosis, and are labeled as stage II and III tumors?

A. Less than 10%
B. 25–30%
C. Approximately 50%
D. Approximately 66%
E. More than 90%

Answer: B. 25–30%

Comment: One-fourth and even up to one-third of all **serous borderline tumors** have spread beyond the ovaries at the time of diagnosis.

Q.20 Expressed in percentages, how many borderline serous tumors are classified as serous surface borderline tumors, i.e. show papillary growth on their external surface?

A. 10%
B. 25–28%
C. 50%
D. 66%
E. >90%

Answer: C. 50%

Comment: Approximately, 50% of all SBTs have papillary structures covering their external surface. These tumors are classified as **serous surface borderline tumors**.

Q.21 A 15 cm ovarian cystic thin walled tumor filled with clear yellow fluid was removed from a 30-year-old woman. The inside surface of the tumor was lined by a single layer of cuboidal to cylindrical cells and scattered ciliated cells. There were no papillae, and there were no signs of nuclear atypia or mitoses. What is the most likely diagnosis?

A. High-grade serous carcinoma
B. Serous cystadenoma
C. Serous borderline tumor
D. Mucinous carcinoma
E. Endometrioid carcinoma

Answer: B. Serous cystadenoma

Comment: This tumor is lined by an epithelial layer that resembles the epithelium of the fallopian tubes. There are no papillae, no atypia and no mitoses and accordingly this benign tumor best classified as **serous cystadenoma**. There is no evidence of malignancy which excludes the diagnosis of carcinoma. Serous cystadenoma must be distinguished from **serous borderline tumors**, which usually contain papillae projecting into the lumen or on their external surface. Microscopically, SBTs show multilayering and piling up of cells as well as nuclear atypia. **Mucinous cystadenomas** are lined by mucin secreting cells. Various cysts, such as epithelial inclusion cysts of the ovary and Müllerian or Wolffian remnant cysts are also in the differential diagnosis, although they rarely attain such a large size.

Q.22 A multilocular cystic tumor filled with serous fluid was removed from the ovary of a 40-year-old woman. It contained numerous solid areas and papillary excrescences inside the cysts and on its external surface. The tumor had the typical microscopic features of a serous borderline tumor but also contained areas as those shown in Figure 4.6. These areas accounted for approximately 5% of the entire tumor. No invasive glandular structures were identified. What is the best diagnosis?

A. High-grade serous carcinoma
B. Serous cystadenoma
C. Serous borderline tumor
D. Serous borderline tumor, micropapillary type
E. Endometrioid carcinoma

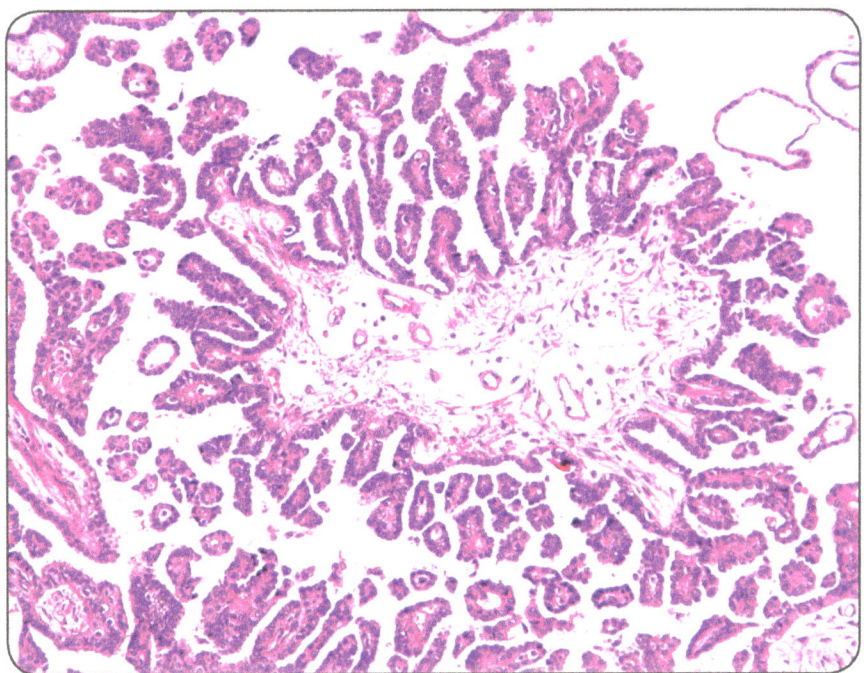

Figure 4.6

Answer: C. Serous borderline tumor

Comment: Up to 10% of all **serous borderline tumors** may contain areas of **micropapillary** growth pattern ("caput medusa like"). If the micropapillary growth pattern does not exceed 10% of the total tumor mass it should not be included in the diagnosis of SBT. If the micropapillary pattern exceeds 10% of the tumor mass, or its foci measure more than 5 mm in diameter, it should be included in the diagnosis (e.g. "SBT, micropapillary type").

Micropapillary growth pattern, is recognized by the characteristic arrangement of thin micropapillae that are five times longer than their cross-sectional diameter, arising abruptly from the central bulbous fibrous core. Micropapillae do not show hierarchical branching and they have no central fibrovascular core.

Contd...

Contd...

Micropapillary SBT must be distinguished from **high-grade serous carcinoma (HGSC) with micropapillary features**, which is diagnosed when the foci of invasion exceed 10 square millimeters or their depth measures more than 5 mm diameter. Most HGSC with micropapillary features show other signs of malignancy and the diagnosis of HGSC is readily made. In questionable cases, the malignancy is best recognized by the presence of deep stromal invasion and foci of necrosis, as well as the formation of vascularized papillae which are wider and irregular, or confluent.

Q.23 What is the most likely diagnosis for this multilocular tumor filled with serous fluid, showing external surface papillary excrescences (Figure 4.7)?

  A. High-grade serous carcinoma
  B. Serous cystadenoma
  C. Serous borderline tumor
  D. Serous borderline tumor, micropapillary type
  E. Endometrioid carcinoma

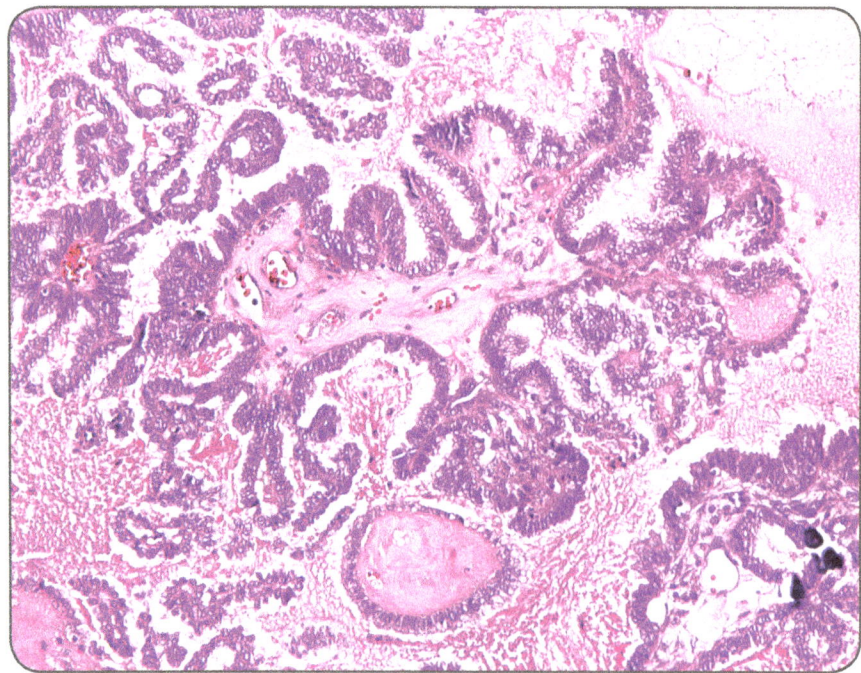

Figure 4.7

Answer: C. Serous borderline tumor

Comment: This tumor is composed of papillae showing hierarchical branching typical of serous borderline tumor.

Q.24 Which cells become especially prominent in serous borderline tumor showing microinvasion of the stroma?

  A. Ciliated cells
  B. Nonciliated columnar cells
  C. Cells showing apocrine secretion
  D. Eosinophilic cells
  E. Mucinous cells

Answer: D. Eosinophilic cells

Comment: Eosinophilic cells are more pronounced in foci of microinvasion.

Q.25 This ovarian multilocular cystic tumor (Figure 4.8) will most likely show immunohistochemically a diffuse positive reaction with all the following antibodies, *except:*

A. Estrogen receptor
B. Cytokeratin 7 (CK7)
C. WT 1
D. p53
E. PAX 8

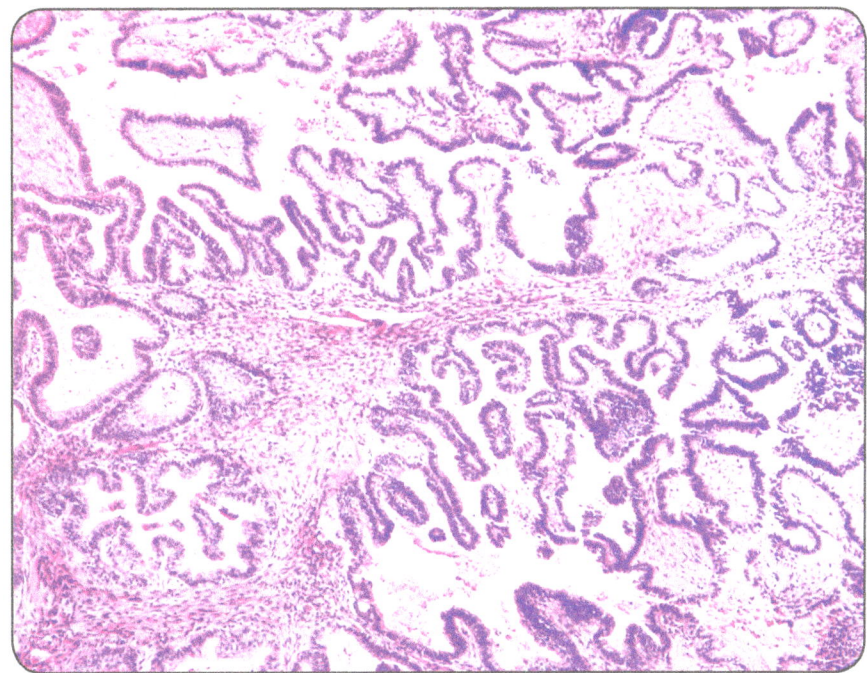

Figure 4.8

Answer: D. p53

Comment: This papillary tumor showing hierarchical branching of its papillae is a **serous borderline tumor**. SBTs do not react **immunohistochemically** with antibodies to p53, although the nuclei of some scattered tumor cells may be weakly positive. In this respect, SBTs differ from high-grade serous carcinomas, which are almost invariably positive for p53. Other antibodies react in a diffusely strong manner with most SBT cells.

Q.26 Genetic studies show that mutations of *BRAF/KRAS* genes are common in all the following tumors, *except:*

A. Serous borderline tumors
B. Serous borderline tumors with micropapillary features
C. Serous borderline tumors with invasive peritoneal metastases
D. Serous cystadenoma adjacent to serous borderline tumor
E. High-grade serous carcinoma

Answer: E. High-grade serous carcinoma

Comment: *BRAF/KRAS* mutations are found in most SBTs, irrespective of their designation. Cystadenoma adjacent to SBT and foci of endosalpingiosis found in these patients also show the same mutations, pointing to a common origin of these lesions. On the other hand *BRAF/KRAS* mutations are not found in high-grade serous carcinomas, pointing out that the histogenesis of these tumors differs from the histogenesis of other, less malignant serous ovarian tumors.

Q.27 What is the recurrence rate of treated serous borderline tumors expressed in percentages?
- A. Less than 5%
- B. 30%
- C. 40–50%
- D. 70%
- E. More than 85%

Answer: C. 40–50%

Comment: Overall **SBT**s have an indolent course but **recurrences** occur in 40–50% cases. Some of these recurrences occur even 10 years after diagnosis. Those with invasive implants have a higher rate or recurrence and also a higher mortality, in contrast to less than 5% mortality of patients who have SBT with noninvasive peritoneal implants. In about 5% of patients with SBTs, there is progression to low-grade serous carcinoma, and most of these patients will usually have invasive implants.

Q.28 Expressed in percentages, how often will the pathologists find benign Müllerian cyst inclusions and/or endosalpingiosis in pelvic and para-aortic lymph nodes removed from patients with serous borderline tumors?
- A. Almost never
- B. 10%
- C. 25%
- D. 50%
- E. In more than 80% cases

Answer: D. 50%

Comment: **Benign Müllerian cyst inclusions and/or endosalpingiosis** are found in pelvic and para-aortic lymph nodes of 50% patients with SBTs. Such inclusions are found only in 10% women who had such lymph node dissection for other reasons.

Q.29 All the following are features of low-grade serous carcinoma, *except:*
- A. Frequently associated with serous borderline components
- B. Marked variation in the size and shape of nuclei
- C. Hyalinized stroma
- D. Psammoma bodies
- E. Rare mitotic figures

Answer: B. Marked variation in the size and shape of nuclei

Comment: **Low-grade serous carcinomas** have small relatively uniform nuclei showing only mild atypia, and no significant anisonucleosis. Variation in size and even moderate nuclear enlargement and atypia, high mitotic count and increased number of MIB-1 positive cells are not found in LGSC. Tumors displaying those features should be classifies as HGSC.

Q.30 The ovarian tumor shown in Figure 4.9 was surgically resected from a 52-year-old woman. Under which heading should this tumor be classified?

A. Serous borderline tumors
B. Serous borderline tumors with noninvasive peritoneal implants
C. Serous borderline tumors with invasive peritoneal implants
D. Low-grade serous carcinomas
E. High-grade serous carcinomas

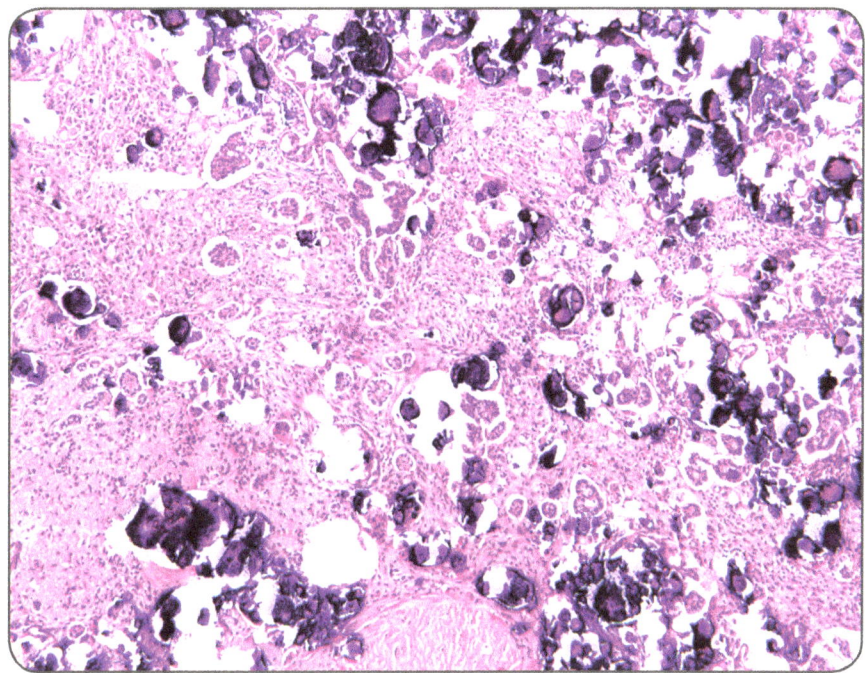

Figure 4.9

Answer: D. Low-grade serous carcinomas

Comment: This tumor contains numerous psammoma bodies and low-grade cells forming short papillae, and is thus classified as a **psammocarcinoma**. This rare ovarian tumor has all the clinical features of **LGSC** and has thus a very good prognosis. Even though most tumors are diagnosed in stage III the long-term survival is almost 95%.

Q.31 Figure 4.10 shows an ovarian tumor resected from a 40-year-old woman known to have a familial germline mutation of *BRCA1*. What is the most appropriate diagnosis?

A. Serous cystadenoma
B. Serous borderline tumor
C. Seromucinous borderline tumor
D. Low-grade serous carcinomas
E. High-grade serous carcinomas

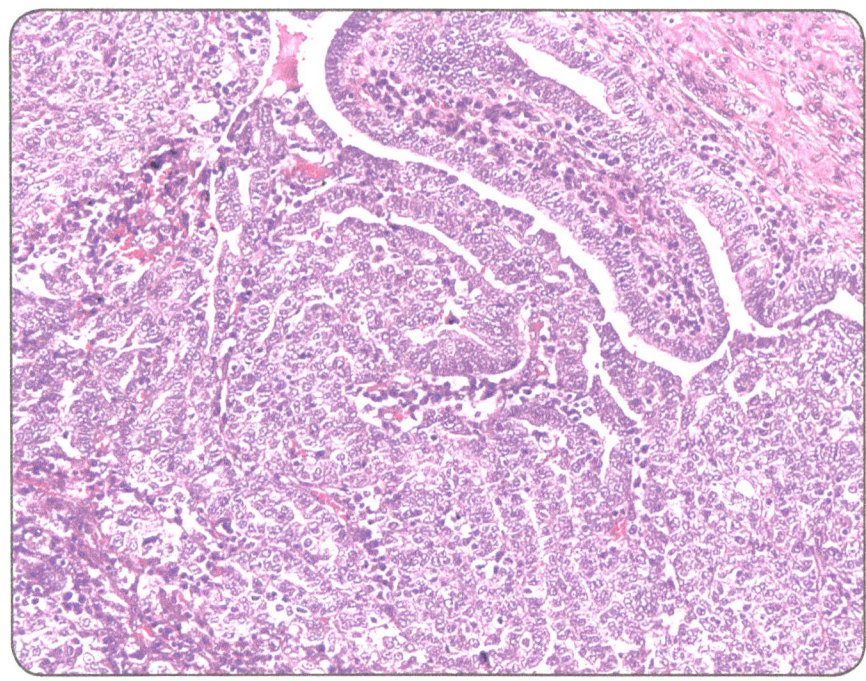

Figure 4.10

Answer: E. High-grade serous carcinomas

Comment: This high-grade serous carcinoma is composed of papillary and solid areas. Women with germline mutations of **BRCA1** or **BRCA2** have a risk of up to 70% of developing ovarian/tubal carcinoma by the age of 70 years and most of these tumors are **HGSC**. Many of these tumors show a **SET growth pattern**, in which the acronym SET stands for solid, endometrioid, and transitional carcinoma (*Source:* Soslow RA, et al. Mod Pathol. 2012; 25: 625-36).

Q.32 The fimbriated part of the fallopian tube of many women with high-grade serous carcinoma of the ovary contains foci of serous intratubal carcinoma (STIC), considered to be potential precursors of the ovarian carcinoma. Antibody to which antigen reacts strongly and diffusely with STIC cells?

A. p53
B. B-RAF
C. K-RAS
D. Calretinin
E. Cytokeratin 5 (CK5)

Answer: A. p53

Comment: **p53** is a good marker for **STIC**, which also shows increased reactivity with antibody **Ki-67 (MIB-1)** in a range from 40 to 95%. Immunoreactivity with the antibody to p53 may be seen in normal fallopian tubes. Foci of at least 12 secretory cells which are p53 positive low Ki-67 reactivity and no nuclear atypia are called "**p53 signature**". At least one-half of these cells show mutations of *TP53* gene, and are considered to be potential precursors of STIC and HGSC.

Q.33 All the following are features of high-grade serous carcinoma, *except:*
   A. High anisonucleosis (nuclear variation exceeding 3 times normal nuclear sizes)
   B. Mitoses in excess of 12 per 10 high power fields
   C. Prominent apoptosis
   D. Prominent necrosis
   E. Coexistence of low-grade serous carcinoma or serous borderline tumor

Answer: E. Coexistence of low-grade serous carcinoma or serous borderline tumor.

Comment: **High-grade serous carcinomas** usually show remarkable uniformity from one field to another. **Coexistent LGSC or SBT** admixed to the HGSC are almost never seen or are found exceptionally rarely.

Q.34 Figure 4.11 was taken from a section of a partially solid ovarian tumor was removed from a 61-year-old woman. This tumor will most likely react immunohistochemically with all the following antibodies except antibodies to which of the following markers?
   A. Cytokeratins 7 (CK 7)   B. WT-1
   C. p16   D. Calretinin
   E. BRCA1

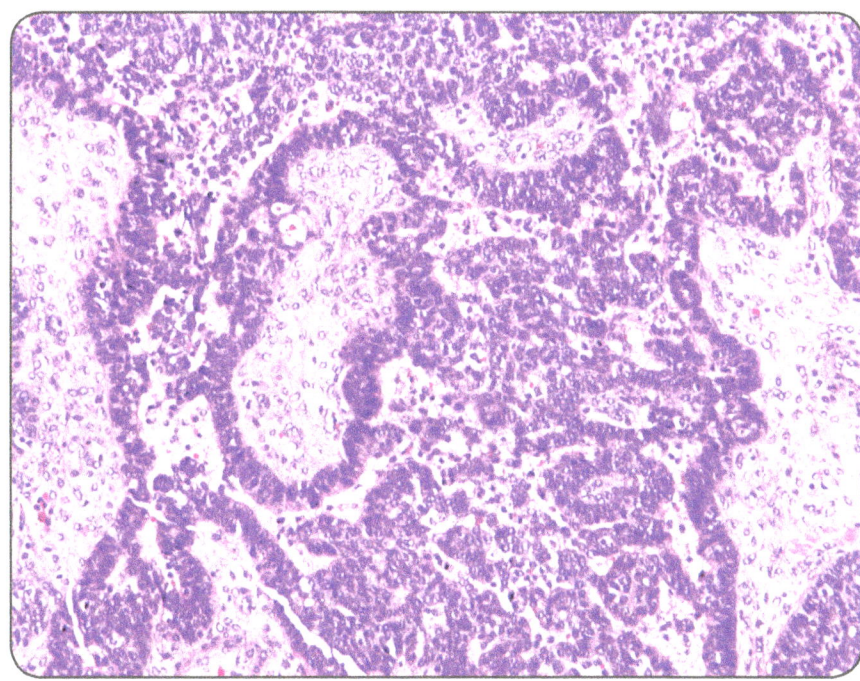

Figure 4.11

Answer: D. Calretinin

Comment: This tumor is a **high-grade serous carcinoma** and it will most likely react with all the antibodies except calretinin, a mesothelial marker which is not expressed in HGSC.

Q.35 What is the most common site of extraperitoneal metastasis of high-grade serous carcinoma?

    A. Lungs
    B. Pleural cavity
    C. Mediastinal lymph nodes
    D. Neck
    E. Brain

Answer: B. Pleural cavity

Comment: **HGSC** tend to metastasize first to the **pleura**, but in later stages of the disease all organs can be reached by hematogenous metastases.

Q.36 Most high-grade serous carcinomas are diagnosed in which FIGO (2014) stage?

    A. IA
    B. II B
    C. III A
    D. III B
    E. III C

Answer: E. III C

Comment: Most **HGSC** are diagnosed in **FIGO (2014) stage III**, i.e. have macroscopic peritoneal metastases beyond the pelvic brim, measuring more than 2 cm in greatest diameter, with or without retroperitoneal lymph node involvement.

Q.37 What is the expected range of 10 year survival of patients treated for FIGO stage II high-grade serous carcinoma, as expressed in percentages?

    A. 80–95%
    B. 60–75%
    C. 50–60%
    D. 30–50%
    E. Less than 30%

Answer: A. 80–95%

Comment: **Ten year survival** of treated stage II patients with HGSC is in the range of 80–95%, in contrast to the survival of patients with stage III and IV HGSC that is less than 30%.

Q.38 Which of the following are the largest ovarian tumors on record?

    A. Serous cystadenomas
    B. Serous borderline tumors
    C. Mucinous cystadenoma and borderline tumors
    D. Low-grade serous carcinomas
    E. Brenner tumors

Answer: C. Mucinous cystadenoma and borderline tumors

Comment: **Mucinous cystadenomas** and **mucinous borderline tumors** may attain a huge size and belong to the largest ovarian tumors on record. It is not unusual to see some of these tumors measuring more than 30 cm in diameter and weighing 20–30 kilograms.

Q.39 A multilocular 10 cm tumor was removed from the right ovary of a 25-year-old woman (Figure 4.12). What is the most likely diagnosis?

A. Serous cystadenoma
B. Serous borderline tumor
C. Seromucinous borderline tumor
D. Low-grade serous carcinomas
E. Mucinous cystadenoma

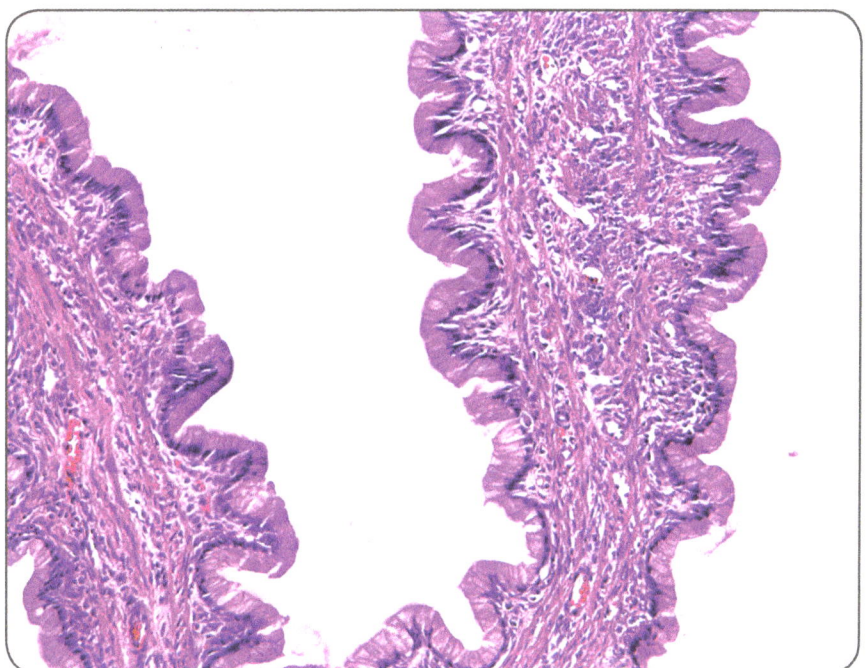

Figure 4.12

Answer: E. Mucinous cystadenoma

Comment: The cystic spaces are lined by benign mucinous cells with basally located nuclei and abound intracytoplasmic mucus, typical of benign **mucinous cystadenoma.**

Q.40 Which of the following statements is true about benign mucinous tumors of the ovary?

A. Most often are unilateral
B. Most often present in form of a unilocular cyst
C. Most often are small (less than 3 cm in diameter)
D. Most have their external surface covered with papillary excrescences
E. Most often are found in women under the age of 20 years

Answer: A. Most often are unilateral

Comment: **Benign mucinous tumors** of the ovary are unilateral in 95% of instances, but a few may be bilateral. They are most often multilocular, and they rarely present as a single mucus filled cyst. Most of them measure 5–10 cm in diameter and have a smooth external surface. Although they may be found in young women under the age of 20 years, most of them are diagnosed in women between 20 and 60 years of age.

Q.41 All the following are features of benign mucinous tumor of the ovary, *except:*
- A. Epithelial proliferation of not more than 25–30% of the entire surface
- B. Formation of papillae
- C. Goblet cells
- D. Neuroendocrine cells
- E. Mitotic activity in the crypt-like invaginations

Answer: A. Epithelial proliferation of not more than 25–30% of the entire surface

Comment: **Epithelial proliferation** of less than 10% of the entire surface is by definition a feature of **benign mucinous tumors**, and all tumors containing more proliferative foci should be classified as borderline. Papillae may are rare in mucinous tumors of the usual intestinal type. All cell types listed here may be seen in benign mucinous tumors, which also may show mitotic activity in their crypt-like invaginations.

Q.42 What is the best diagnosis for this mucinous ovarian tumor (Figure 4.13)?
- A. Serous cystadenoma
- B. Serous borderline tumor
- C. Seromucinous borderline tumor
- D. Mucinous borderline tumor/atypical proliferative mucinous tumor
- E. Mucinous cystadenoma

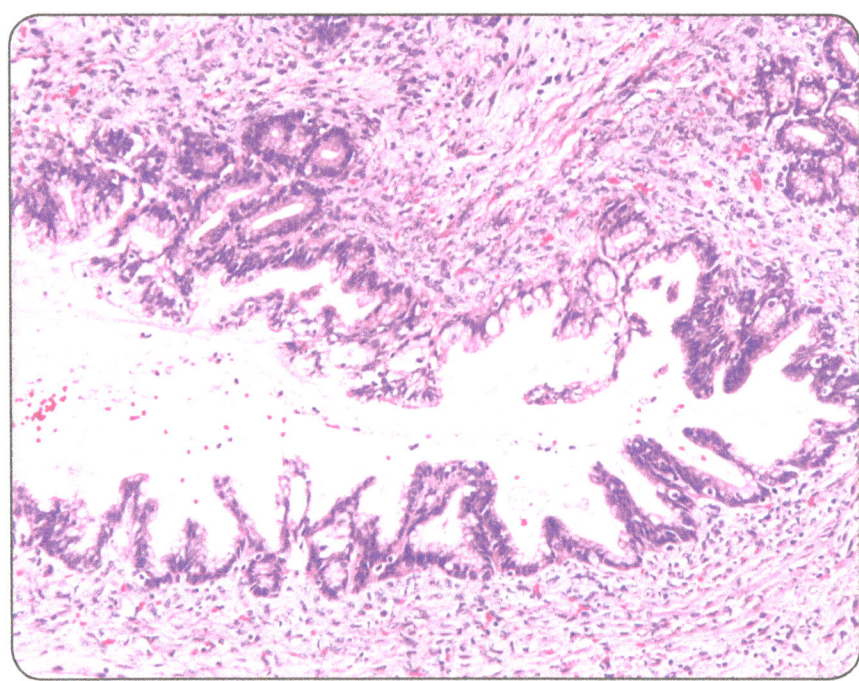

Figure 4.13

Answer: D. Mucinous borderline tumor/atypical proliferative mucinous tumor

Comment: This mucinous epithelium shows focal proliferative stratitification and formation of slender papillae, as well as grouping of glands. Nuclear atypia can be surmised from the darker staining of hyperchromatic cells. All these findings are consistent with the diagnosis of **mucinous borderline tumor/atypical proliferative mucinous tumor (MBT/APMT).** These tumors account for 30–50% of ovarian borderline tumors in North America and Europe and for 70% of such tumors in Asia.

Q.43 Figure 4.14 shows a lesion identified in the stromal part of a benign mucinous tumor of the ovary. What is the most appropriate diagnosis?

A. Dermoid cyst
B. Mesothelioma
C. Squamous metaplasia of endometriosis
D. Transitional carcinoma
E. Brenner tumor

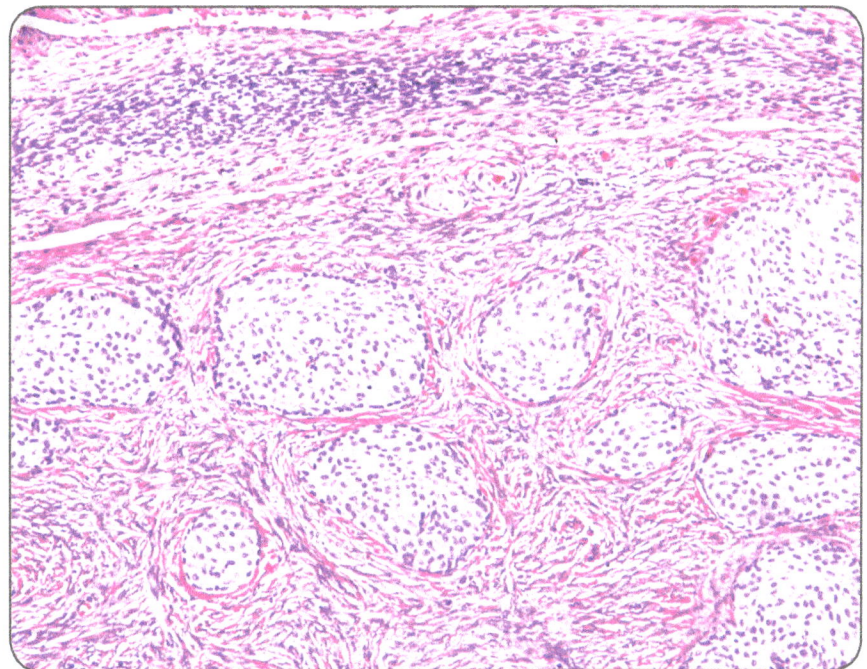

Figure 4.14

Answer: E. Brenner tumor

Comment: **Brenner tumor** is found in 15–20% of **benign mucinous tumor** of the ovary. Dermoid cysts also may be found but less often (in 3–5% cases). Molecular biology studies have shown that the Brenner tumor component is monoclonal with the mucinous component in such tumors, indicating a common origin (*Source:* Wang Y, et al. J Pathol. 2015;237:146–151).

Q.44 Hormonal symptoms in women with ovarian mucinous tumors are related to secretion of steroids from which cells?

A. Adjacent ovarian stroma
B. Stroma of the tumor
C. Mucinous cells
D. Neuroendocrine cells
E. Inflammatory cells reacting to extravasated mucus

Answer: A. Adjacent ovarian stroma

Comment: Increased cellularity of the adjacent **ovarian stroma**, often associated with focal luteinization of stromal cells is common in the vicinity of ovarian **mucinous tumors**, accounting for hypersecretion of steroid hormones. Mucinous tumors are actually the most common nonendocrine tumors of the ovary causing **endocrine symptoms**.

Q.45 Mucin filled unilocular cystic tumors, each measuring 10 cm in diameter, were removed from the ovaries of a 30-year-old woman who also had endometriosis. Tumors were diagnosed as borderline seromucinous tumors. Which of the following features is typically seen microscopically in all such tumors?

A. Goblet cells
B. Neuroendocrine cells
C. Complex papillae showing hierarchical branching
D. Infiltrates of plasma cells and lymphocytes in the stroma of the papillae
E. Destructive stromal invasion 10 mm in diameter

Answer: C. Complex papillae showing hierarchical branching

Comment: Complex papillae similar to those in SBT are commonly seen in **seromucinous borderline tumors**, which were previously known as **borderline mucinous tumors of endocervical type**. These tumors differ from BMT of the intestinal type, which have thinner papillae with filiform branching. Goblet cells and neuroendocrine cells are not seen in seromucinous tumors. The columnar epithelium is of the endocervical type. In addition to serous, ciliated, and mucinous cells one may find foci of endometrioid glands with squamous metaplasia, consistent with the Müllerian origin of such tumors. Foci of adjacent endometriosis also favor the Müllerian origin of these tumors. Infiltrates of inflammatory cells in the fibrous cores of the papillae contain inflammatory cells but those are typically neutrophils rather than plasma cells and lymphocytes. Microinvasion up to 5 mm may be present but larger destructive invasion is not a feature of these tumors, but rather a sign of truly invasive carcinoma. Seromucinous carcinomas are uncommon (*Source:* Taylor J, McCluggage WG. Am J Surg Pathol. 2015; 39:983-92).

Q.46 Bilateral ovarian tumors were found in a 55-year-old woman. The tumors were partially cystic and partially solid. Figure 4.15 shows the typical histologic findings, which are representative of both ovarian tumors. Tumor cells were CDX2 and CK20 positive. What is the most likely diagnosis?

A. Serous cystadenoma
B. Mucinous cystadenoma
C. Low-grade serous carcinoma
D. Mucinous adenocarcinoma
E. Metastasis from a colonic adenocarcinoma

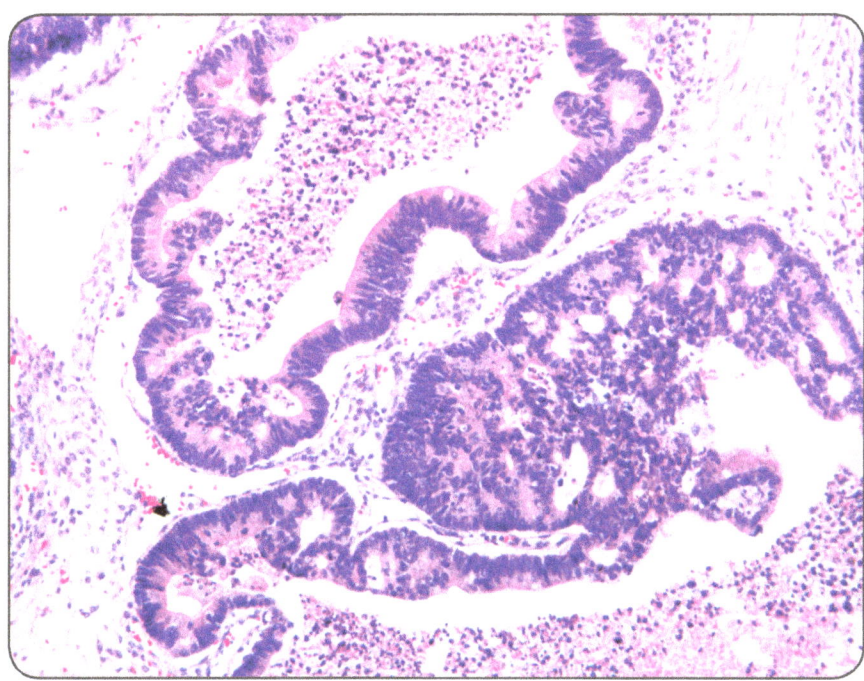

Figure 4.15

Answer: **E. Metastasis from a colonic adenocarcinoma**

Comment: Figure 4.15 forms garland-like and cribriform structures with prominent areas of "dirty necrosis", most consistent with **metastases from a colonic primary**. Positive immunoreactivity with the antibodies to CDX2 and CK20 supports the diagnosis.

Q.47 When examining a mucinous adenocarcinomas of the ovary, all the following findings favor a metastasis from the lower gastrointestinal tract over a primary ovarian mucinous carcinoma, *except:*

   A. Bilateral tumors
   B. Small tumors measuring less than 10 cm in largest diameter, solid but oozing mucus on cross-sectioning
   C. Coexistence of cystadenoma/borderline mucinous tumor and carcinoma in the same mass
   D. Cytokeratin immunoprofile CK7-/CK20+
   E. Presence of pseudomyxoma peritonei

Answer: **C. Coexistence of cystadenoma/borderline mucinous tumor and carcinoma in the same mass**

Comment: Most primary **ovarian mucinous carcinomas** evolve often from pre-existing benign mucinous cystadenoma or BMT, both of which may be found in the same tumor mass. **Coexisting cystadenoma and invasive mucinous adenocarcinoma** favor the diagnosis of a primary ovarian tumor.

Bilateral tumors, especially if small and mostly solid or those associated with pseudomyxoma peritonei favor the diagnosis of a primary colonic adenocarcinoma with metastases to the ovary. Immunoprofile CK7-/CK20+ is typical of primary colonic adenocarcinoma and is preserved in tumors, which have metastasized to the ovary. However, metastases to the ovary may show significant variation in the expression of antigens considered to be typical of lower GI tract, and thus, one should be cautious when interpreting the immunohistochemical data.

Factors favoring the diagnosis of primary ovarian mucinous carcinoma versus a metastasis from the lower GI tract are listed in the Table 4.2.

Table 4.2: Features favoring the diagnosis of primary ovarian mucinous carcinoma versus metastasis from the lower gastrointestinal tract

Feature	Favoring primary ovarian mucinous carcinoma	Favoring metastases from the lower gastrointestinal tract
Coexistent benign cystadenoma or MBT in the tumor mass	++	
Bilateral tumors*#		++
Small size of tumors (<10 cm)#		++
Multinodular solid growth		++
Surface implants on the ovary		++
Tumor growth predominantly in the hilum and mesovarium		++
Pseudomyxoma ovarii (mucus in the stroma of the ovary)		++
Extraovarian tumor or pseudomyxoma peritonei *		++
Expansile (confluent) microscopic growth pattern without destructive stromal invasion	++	
Complex papillary growth pattern microscopically	++	
Signet ring cell prominence in microscopic sections		++
Immunoprofile CK7-/CK20+		++

Abbreviations: MBT, mucinous borderline tumor; CK, cytokeratin.
* Most ovarian mucinous adenocarcinomas (80%) are unilateral and stage I, and are not accompanied by extraovarian seeding or masses
# A note of caution: Up to 40% of metastases from the lower GI tract are unilateral and measure more than 10 in diameter
Source: Mutter GL, Prat J (Eds). Pathology of the Female Reproductive Tract, 3rd edition. Churchill Livingstone: Elsevier; 2014.

Q.48 A mucinous adenocarcinoma of the ovary was found to be immunohistochemically strongly positive for CK7, p16, and cytoplasmic CEA. The tumor was negative for CK20, vimentin, estrogen and progesterone receptors. What is the most likely diagnosis?

    A. Primary ovarian mucinous adenocarcinoma
    B. Metastatic adenocarcinoma from a colonic primary
    C. Metastatic carcinoma from a pancreatic primary
    D. Metastatic carcinoma from a cervical primary
    E. Metastatic carcinoma from an endometrial primary

Answer: D. Metastatic carcinoma from a cervical primary

Comment: **Cervical mucinous adenocarcinoma** is usually positive for CK7, p16 and cytoplasmic CEA. These tumors are usually negative for CK20, vimentin, estrogen, and progesterone receptors.

Q.49 What is the best diagnosis for the ovarian adenocarcinoma shown in Figure 4.16?

    A. Low-grade serous carcinoma
    B. High-grade serous carcinoma
    C. Mucinous cystadenoma
    D. Clear cell carcinoma
    E. Endometrioid carcinoma

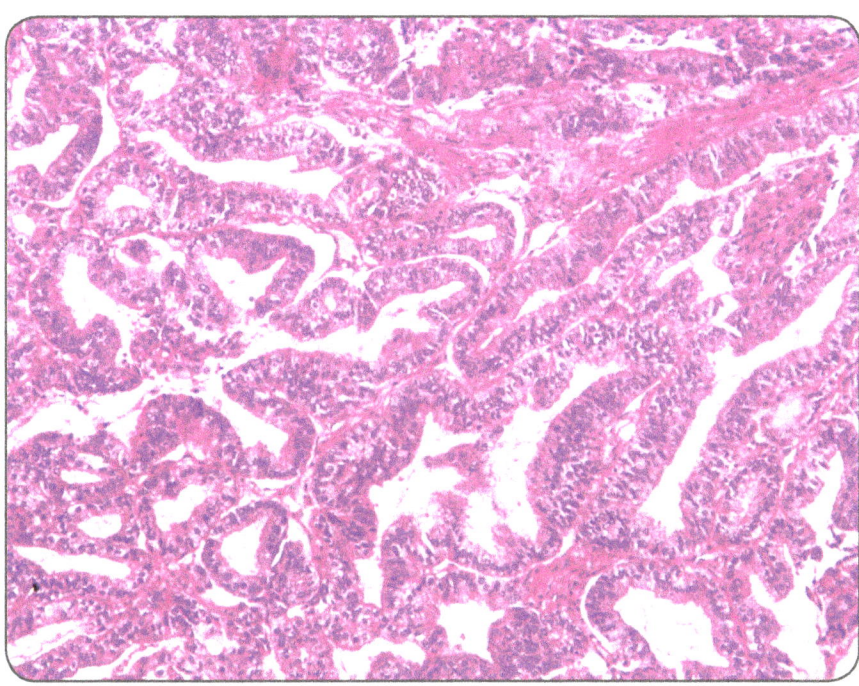

Figure 4.16

Answer: E. Endometrioid carcinomas

Comment: The **endometrioid carcinoma** shown in Figure 4.16 is composed of glands lined by cylindrical cells with oval or elongated nuclei resembling a low-grade endometrial adenocarcinoma of the uterus.

Q.50 What is the best diagnosis for the solid ovarian tumor removed from a 55-year-old woman (Figure 4.17)?

    A. Endometrioid adenocarcinoma   B. Serous adenofibroma
    C. Endometriosis   D. Serous borderline tumor
    E. Brenner tumor, cystic

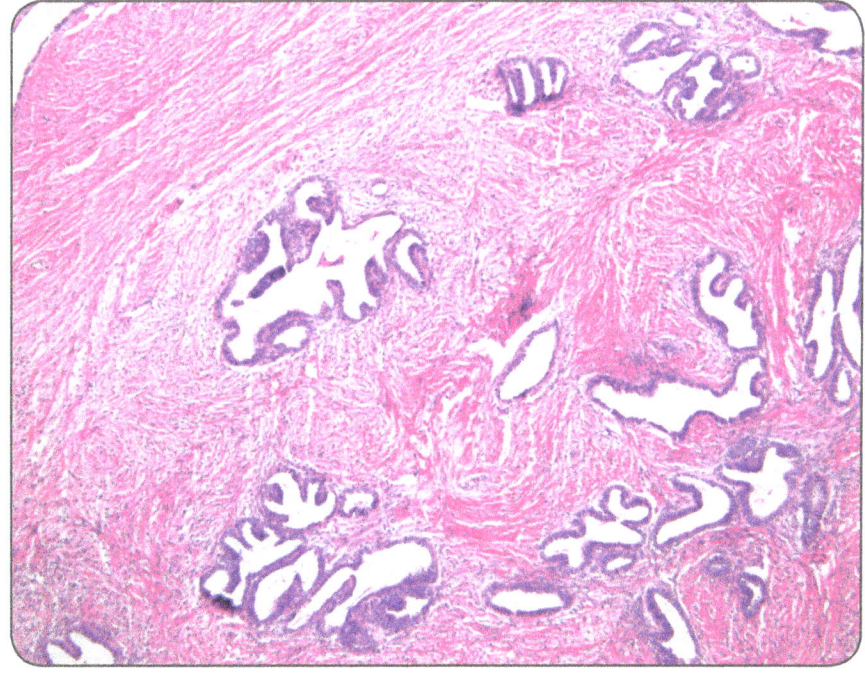

Figure 4.17

Answer: B. Serous adenofibroma

Comment: Figure 4.17 shows an **adenofibroma**, i.e. a tumor composed of abundant fibrous stroma surrounding scattered "benign" glands lined by a one cell thick cuboidal epithelium. At higher magnification, the lining of glands resembled the epithelium of fallopian tubes and thus it was classified as **serous adenofibroma**. If the epithelium were endometrial-like, it would have been classified as **endometrioid adenofibroma**. In some adenofibromas, the glands are line by mucinous epithelium and in some others by clear cell epithelium; they are named accordingly **mucinous or clear cell adenofibromas**. Such minor differences in the appearance of the glandular lining have no clinical significance.

It should be noticed that some adenofibromas may show signs of incipient malignancy and are then classified as borderline tumors. Endometrioid adenofibromas are considered to be the rare benign equivalents of endometrioid adenocarcinoma of the ovary. Borderline endometrioid adenofibromas are even less common than benign endometrioid adenofibromas.

Q.51 Approximately 15–20% of primary ovarian carcinomas are associated with uterine endometrial adenocarcinoma. What is the predominant microscopic type of ovarian cancer in such cases?

- A. Low-grade serous carcinoma
- B. High-grade serous carcinoma
- C. Mucinous cystadenocarcinoma
- D. Clear cell carcinoma
- E. Endometrioid carcinoma

Answer: E. Endometrioid carcinoma

Comment: In most cases, these endometrial and ovarian malignancies develop simultaneously and are both low-grade **endometrioid carcinomas**. Following hystero-salpingoophorectomy the five-year survival rate of patients with ovarian endometrioid carcinoma is 70–90%. Both tumors usually show the same type of *PTEN* mutation.

Q.52 What is the most common microscopic growth pattern of ovarian clear cell carcinoma?

- A. Tubulocystic and papillary
- B. Solid
- C. Cribriform
- D. Reticular
- E. Nesting

Answer: A. Tubulocystic and papillary

Comment: **Clear cell carcinomas of the ovary** often have a rather variegated microscopic appearance and thus, it is not uncommon to find several **growth patterns**. The most common combination includes a tubulocystic and a papillary growth pattern. The stroma of these papillae is usually hyalinized.

Q.53 What are the most common cell types in clear cell carcinoma?

- A. Clear polygonal or cuboidal and hobnail cells
- B. Flattened cuboidal cells
- C. Eosinophilic cells forming nests
- D. Signet ring cells arranged in rows or nests
- E. Cylindrical oxyphilic cells

Answer: A. Clear polygonal or cuboidal and hobnail cells

Ovary

Q.54 What is the best diagnosis for the ovarian carcinoma shown in Figure 4.18?

   A. Low-grade serous carcinoma
   B. High-grade serous carcinoma
   C. Mucinous carcinoma
   D. Clear cell carcinoma
   E. Endometrioid carcinoma

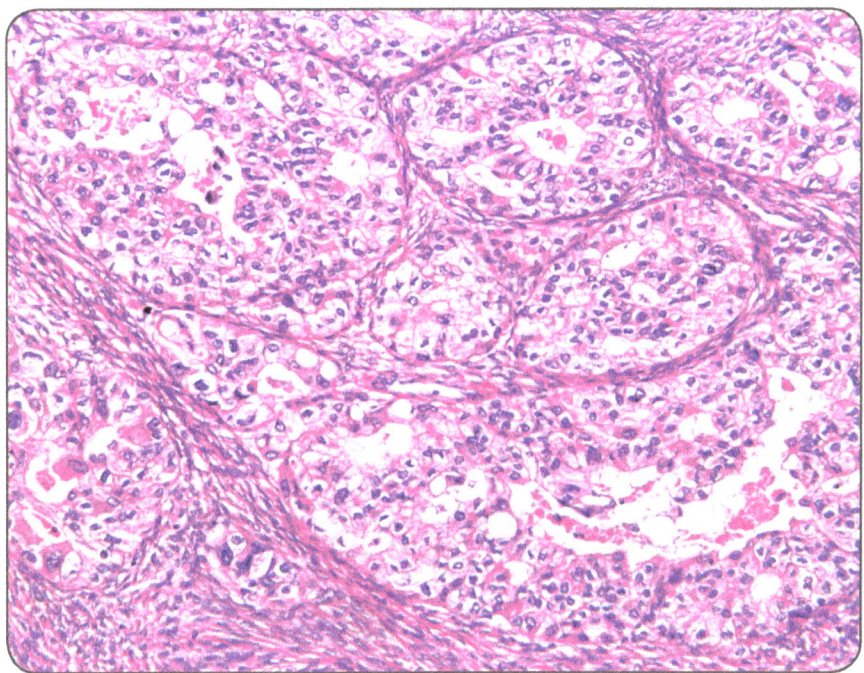

Figure 4.18

Answer: D. Clear cell carcinoma

Comment: Figure 4.18 shows the solid growth pattern of a clear cell carcinoma. Some solid nests have central lumina suggesting abortive gland formation. The cells have hyperchromatic nuclei surrounded by clear cytoplasm and sharp cell membranes.

Q.55 Which ovarian carcinoma is clinically most often associated with paraneoplastic hypercalcemia and thromboembolism?

   A. Low-grade serous carcinomas
   B. High-grade serous carcinomas
   C. Mucinous carcinoma
   D. Endometrioid carcinoma
   E. Clear cell carcinoma

Answer: E. Clear cell carcinoma

Comment: Up to 10% of all cases of paraneoplastic **hypercalcemia** and up to 40% cases of **venous thromboses** related to ovarian cancers are associated with **clear cell carcinoma**. Women with clear cell carcinoma have a 2.5 times higher chance for venous thrombosis than those with other forms of ovarian cancer.

Q.56 What is the best diagnosis for the ovarian carcinoma shown in Figure 4.19?
  A. Low-grade serous carcinoma
  B. High-grade serous carcinoma
  C. Mucinous carcinoma
  D. Clear cell carcinoma
  E. Endometrioid carcinoma

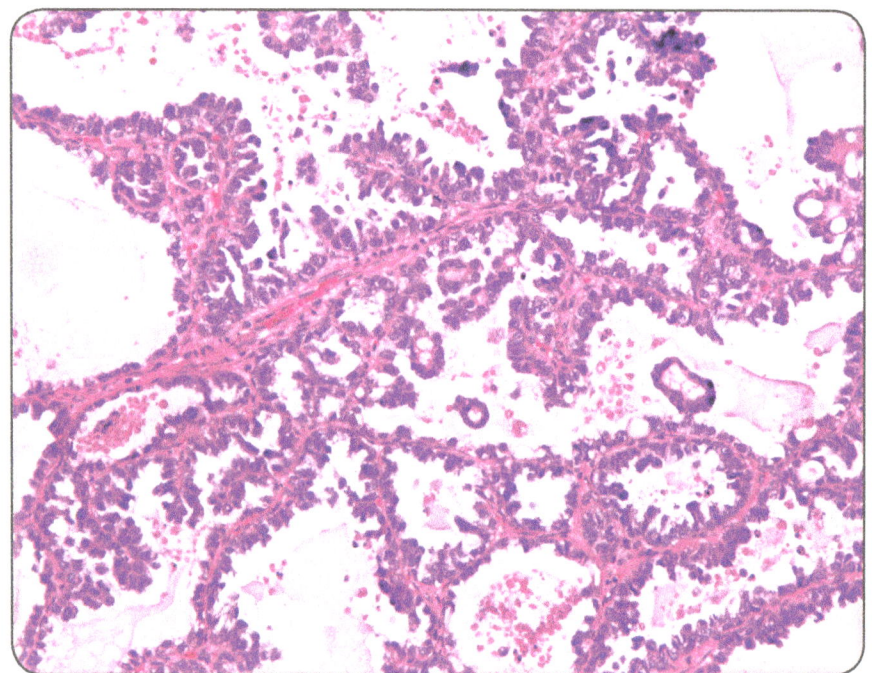

Figure 4.19

Answer: D. Clear cell carcinoma

Comment: Figure 4.19 shows a **tubulocystic clear cell carcinoma** of the ovary. Even at this low magnification one may see the hobnail appearance of tumor cells lining dilated tubular structures and a few short papillae projecting into their lumens.

Q.57 Antibodies to which of the following antigens have the highest sensitivity and specificity for ovarian clear cell carcinoma?
  A. Wilms tumor-1 (WT-1)
  B. Hepatocyte nuclear factor-1 beta
  C. p53
  D. Thyroid transcription factor-1(TTF-1)
  E. Estrogen receptor

Answer: B. Hepatocyte nuclear factor-1 beta

Comment: The high sensitivity and specificity of **hepatocyte nuclear factor-1 beta** is useful for distinguishing clear cell carcinoma from HGSC which is typically negative for this marker and positive for p53, WT-1 and estrogen receptor. Clear cell carcinomas are negative for p53 and estrogen receptor and only sometimes positive for WT-1 (10%) or TTF-1 (less than 20%). HGSC with clear cells are also negative for hepatocyte nuclear factor-1 beta indicating that they are actually serous rather than clear cell carcinomas (*Source:* DeLair D, et al. Int J Gynecol Pathol. 2014; 32: 541-6).

Contd...

Contd...

Unfortunately, this marker is positive in Krukenberg tumors. To separate clear cell from Krukenberg tumors it is thus best to use antibodies to napsin A, which react with clear cell carcinoma, but not with Krukenberg tumors (*Source:* Li Q, et al. Int J Clin Exp Pathol. 2015; 8:8305-10).

Q.58 What is the best diagnosis for the 5 cm ovarian tumor shown in Figure 4.20?
   A. Low-grade serous carcinomas
   B. Brenner tumor
   C. Transitional cell carcinoma
   D. Clear cell carcinoma
   E. Walthard nests

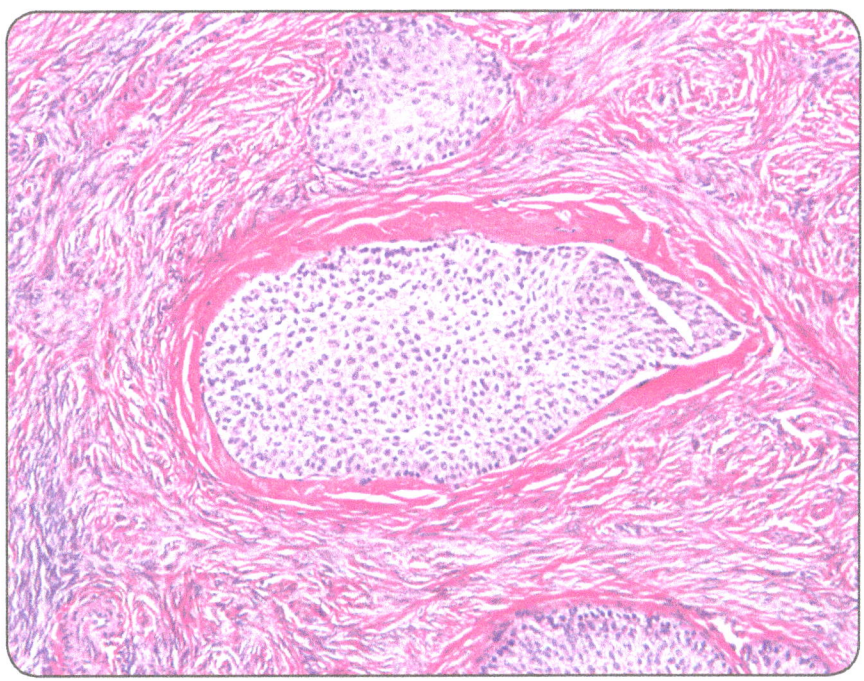

Figure 4.20

Answer: B. Brenner tumor

Comment: This **Brenner tumor** is composed of nests of transitional epithelium showing no atypia and no evidence of invasiveness. **Walthard nests** are microscopic developmental remnants composed of transitional epithelium, usually found in the periovarian soft tissues; they do not form visible tumors.

Q.59 What is the best diagnosis for the ovarian tumor shown in Figure 4.21?
   A. Low-grade serous carcinomas
   B. Brenner tumor
   C. Transitional cell carcinoma
   D. Adenosquamous carcinoma
   E. Clear cell carcinoma

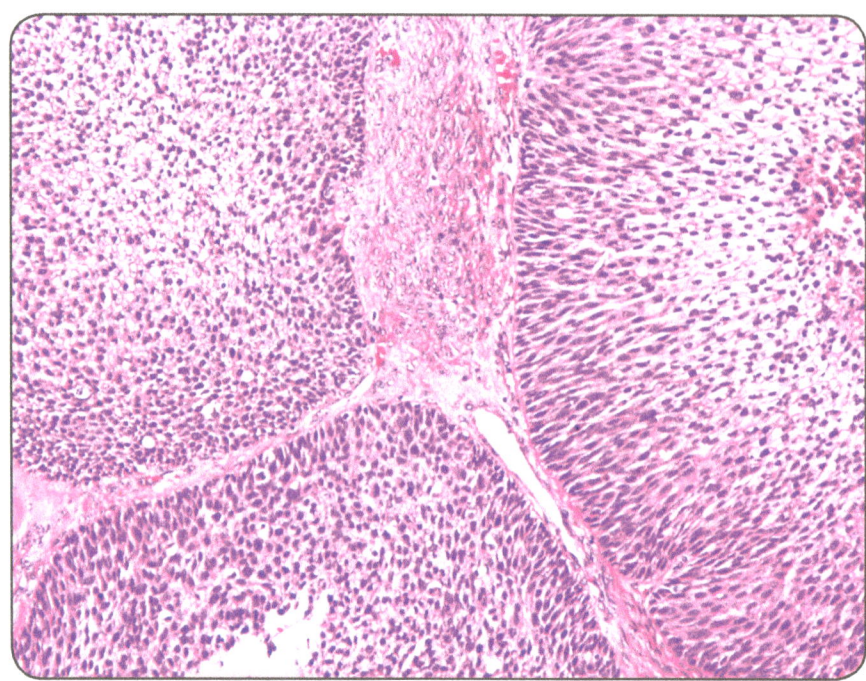

Figure 4.21

Answer: B. Brenner tumor

Comment: The tumor is composed of nests of transitional epithelium showing no atypia. It can be readily distinguished from **transitional cell carcinoma**, a high-grade malignant tumor, currently considered to be a variant of high-grade serous carcinoma.

Q.60 Which one of these immunohistochemical findings favors the diagnosis of malignant Brenner tumor over transitional-like high-grade serous carcinoma?

    A. p53+
    B. WT1+
    C. Estrogen receptor+
    D. p16+
    E. GATA 3+

Answer: E. GATA 3+

Comment: **GATA 3** is a reliable marker of transitional epithelium and it is expressed in essentially all benign and borderline **Brenner tumors** and **most malignant Brenner tumors** tested so far. The other markers are expressed in high-grade transitional-like carcinomas (also known as high-grade transitional carcinomas), currently classified as variants of HGSC.

Q.61 Yolk sac carcinoma of the ovary in women above the age of 40 usually originate from which cells, tissues or pre-existent tumors?

    A. Oocytes
    B. Cortical stroma of the ovary
    C. Teratomas
    D. Dysgerminomas
    E. Epithelial tumors

Answer: E. Epithelial tumors

Comment: Yolk sac carcinoma of the ovary in older women most often originates from epithelial tumors. Less often they originate from teratomas (*Source:* McNamee T, et al. Histopathology. 2016; 69: 739-51).

Q.62 A small papillary cystadenoma was found in the ovary of a 30-year-old woman. It was composed of clear cells lining branching papillae which projected into the lumen of the cyst. This benign tumor is typical of which syndrome?

A. Gardner syndrome
B. Muir-Torre syndrome
C. von Hippel-Lindau syndrome
D. Lynch syndrome
E. Peutz-Jeghers syndrome

Answer: **C. von Hippel-Lindau syndrome**

Comment: **Clear cell papillary cystadenoma of the ovary** of patients with **von Hippel-Lindau syndrome** is the female equivalent of this tumor previously described in the epididymis. It is a rare tumor but still not so rare as not to be included in the latest 2014 WHO "blue book" on gynecological tumors.

Q.63 What is the most common undifferentiated small cell carcinoma of the ovary in women under the age of 40 years?

A. Small cell undifferentiated carcinoma, hypercalcemic type
B. Small cell carcinoma, pulmonary type
C. Small cell carcinoma, nonpulmonary type
D. Transitional-like carcinoma
E. High-grade serous carcinoma

Answer: **A. Small cell undifferentiated carcinoma, hypercalcemic type.**

Comment: Small cell undifferentiated carcinoma, hypercalcemic type is a rare tumor, yet it is the most common undifferentiated carcinoma in younger women under the age of 40 years.

Q.64 What is the most common sex cord-stromal tumor of the ovary?

A. Granulosa cell tumor
B. Fibroma
C. Sertoli-Leydig cell tumor
D. Sclerosing stromal tumor
E. Thecoma

Answer: **B. Fibroma**

Comment: Fibroma is the most common tumor of this group, accounting for 4% of all ovarian tumors, whereas thecomas account for 1% (Kurman et al. 2014). The data from the 25 years' files of Massachusetts General Hospital, cited in the book of Mutter and Prat (2014), indicate that 87% sex cord-stromal tumors belonged to the thecoma-fibroma group. Granulosa cell tumors comprised 12%, whereas all others accounted for less than 1% of sex cord-stromal and steroid tumors of the ovary.

Q.65 Which of the following is the most common sex cord-stromal ovarian tumor associated with clinical signs of hyperestrinism?

A. Adult granulosa cell tumor
B. Juvenile granulosa cell tumor
C. Sclerosing stromal tumor
D. Thecoma
E. Fibroma

Answer: A. Adult granulosa cell tumor

Comment: Granulosa tumors account for approximately 75% of all ovarian tumors associated with estrogenic symptoms.

Q.66 Which of the following sex cord-stromal tumors is most often associated with virilization?
  A. Adult granulosa cell tumor
  B. Juvenile granulosa cell tumor
  C. Thecoma
  D. Sertoli-Leydig cell tumor
  E. Fibroma

Answer: D. Sertoli-Leydig cell tumor

Comment: Between 40% and 60% of all patients with **Sertoli-Leydig cell tumors** (SLCT) show signs of virilization. In some patients, SLCTs secrete estrogens and some are hormonally inactive.

Q.67 What is the best diagnosis for the ovarian sex-cord stromal tumors shown in Figure 4.22?
  A. Thecoma
  B. Adult granulosa cell tumor
  C. Juvenile granulosa cell tumor
  D. Gynandroblastoma
  E. Sclerosing stromal tumor

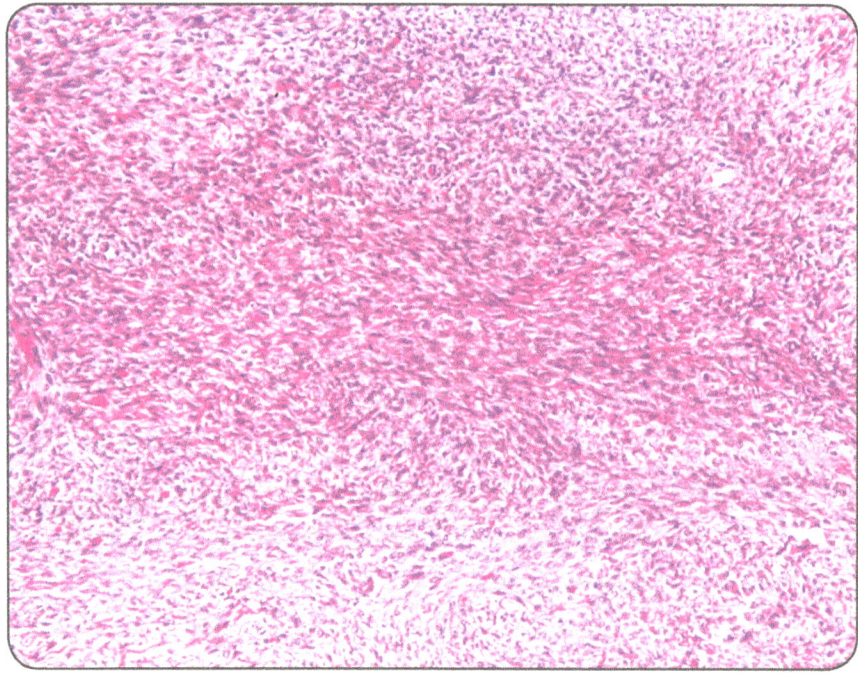

Figure 4.22

Answer: A. Thecoma

Comment: Figure 4.22 shows a benign tumor composed of sheets of uniform cells with oval or round nuclei and pale cytoplasm with ill-defined borders.

Q.68 **Which one the following sex cord-stromal tumors has the highest chance of recurrence?**
- A. Adult granulosa cell tumor
- B. Juvenile granulosa cell tumor
- C. Fibroma
- D. Thecoma
- E. Sclerosing stromal tumor

Answer: **A. Adult granulosa cell tumor**

Comment: **Adult granulosa cell tumors** are low-grade malignant tumors with an overall recurrence rate up to 30%. Even early stage I tumors recur at a rate of 10–15%. All other tumors listed in this question are usually benign and as a rule do not recur.

Q.69 **Which of the following tumors has angular and coffee-bean-shaped grooved nuclei and contains Call-Exner bodies?**
- A. Adult granulosa cell tumor
- B. Juvenile granulosa cell tumor
- C. Fibroma
- D. Steroid-cell tumor
- E. Thecoma

Answer: **A. Adult granulosa cell tumor**

Comment: The nuclei of **adult granulosa cell tumors** are angulated or coffee-bean-shaped and often grooved. In the microfollicular growth pattern, tumor cells form Call-Exner bodies, but these are found in less than one-half of all tumors.

Q.70 **What is the most common microscopic growth pattern of adult granulosa cell tumors?**
- A. Diffuse
- B. Microfollicular
- C. Macrofollicular
- D. Gyriform
- E. Insular

Answer: **A. Diffuse**

Comment: Diffuse growth pattern, characterized by no recognizable pattern, is present in more than one-half of all **adult granulosa cell tumors**. Other, more characteristic patterns, are however usually admixed to the predominant pattern, allowing for an easier identification of these tumors as adult granulose cell tumors.

Q.71 **What is the best diagnosis for the ovarian sex-cord stromal tumors shown in Figure 4.23?**
- A. Thecoma
- B. Adult granulosa cell tumor
- C. Juvenile granulosa cell tumor
- D. Gynandroblastoma
- E. Sclerosing stromal tumor

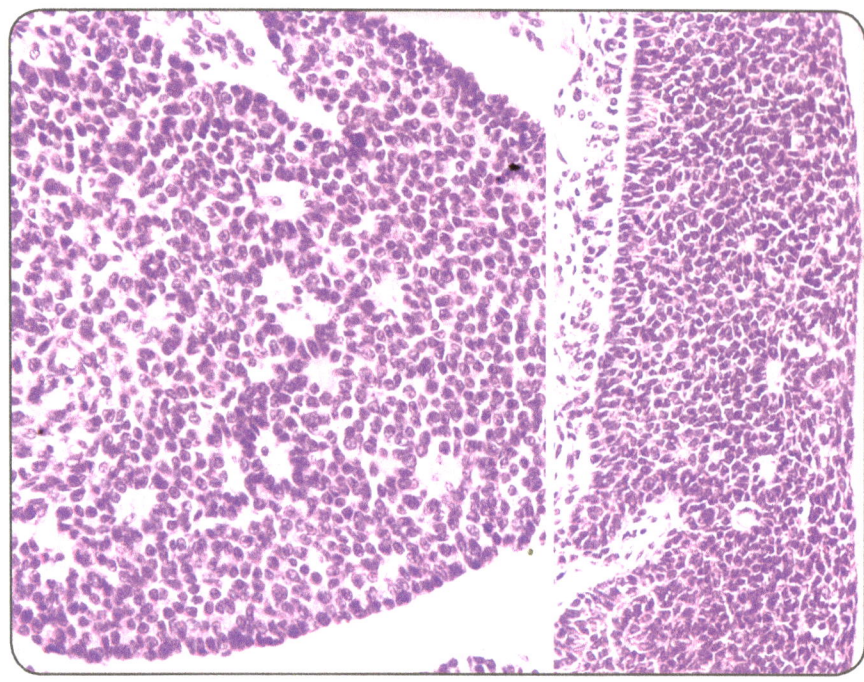

Figure 4.23

Answer: B. Adult granulosa cells tumor

Comment: Figure 4.23 shows a microfollicular **granulosa cell tumor** with numerous Call-Exner bodies.

Q.72 Antibody to which of the following cell markers typically reacts with adult granulosa cell tumors?
- A. α-inhibin
- B. Cytokeratin CK7
- C. Cytokeratin CK20
- D. Epithelial membrane antigen
- E. Thyroid transcription factor 1

Answer: A. α-inhibin

Comment: **α-inhibin** is a good marker for all ovarian **sex cord-stromal and steroid cell tumors** including **granulosa cell tumors**. The antibodies to other markers listed here are unreactive with adult granulosa cell tumors.

Q.73 Reticulin stain demonstrates pericellular reticulin fibers in all the following tumors, *except:*
- A. Fibroma
- B. Thecoma
- C. Adult granulosa cell tumor
- D. Endometrial stromal sarcoma
- E. Leiomyoma

Answer: C. Adult granulosa cell tumor

Comment: **Reticulin stain** is useful for distinguishing **adult granulosa cell tumors** from other tumors listed here, which contain stainable pericellular reticulin fibers. Reticulin stain applied to granulosa cell tumor outlines reticulin fibers surrounding groups of cells.

Q.74 All the following features of adult granulosa cell tumors are considered positive predictors for recurrence, *except:*
- A. Advanced stage of the tumor
- B. Tumor size over 15 cm in diameter
- C. Bilaterality
- D. Tumor rupture
- E. Diffuse growth pattern with high mitotic activity

Answer: **E. Diffuse growth pattern with high mitotic activity**

Comment: Advanced stage is the best predictor for recurrence of **adult granulosa cell tumor**. Large tumor size, bilaterality and tumor rupture are also predictive of recurrence. Histologic findings, including the recognition of several microscopic subtypes of granulosa cell tumors and a high mitotic count have no prognostic significance.

Q.75 Which of the following sex cord-stromal tumors will most likely may secrete alpha fetoprotein into the blood?
- A. Sclerosing stromal tumor
- B. Thecoma
- C. Adult granulosa cell tumor
- D. Endometrial stromal sarcoma
- E. Sertoli-Leydig cell tumor

Answer: **E. Sertoli-Leydig cell tumor**

Comment: In about 20% patients with Sertoli-Leydig cell tumors there is an elevation of serum AFP (*Source:* Gagnon S, et al. Mod Pathol. 1989; 2: 63).

Q.76 All the fallowing statements are true about most juvenile granulosa cell tumors (JGCT), *except:*
- A. JGCT secrete estrogens
- B. JGCT are found in the first decade of life
- C. JGCT cause precocious puberty
- D. JGCT are limited to the ovary and never metastasize
- E. JGCT are solid or predominantly solid containing scattered small cysts

Answer: **C. JGCT cause precocious puberty**

Comment: Most JGCT secrete estrogens which cause **isosexual pseudopuberty**, rather than true **precocious puberty**. These girls have no menstruation because they do not ovulate. Hyperestrinism will, namely, suppress the secretion of pituitary gonadotropins, and without a rise of LH no ovulation will occur. Most JGCT are solid masses or mostly solid, limited to the ovary and found in girls younger than 10 years of age.

Q.77 Figure 4.24 shows the microscopic features of a 7 cm ovarian tumor which was removed from a 60-year-old woman. On cross-section it was solid and yellowish. It was positively stained with Oil-red O. What is the most likely diagnosis?

  A. Fibroma
  B. Thecoma
  C. Adult granulosa cell tumor
  D. Endometrial stromal sarcoma
  E. Leiomyoma

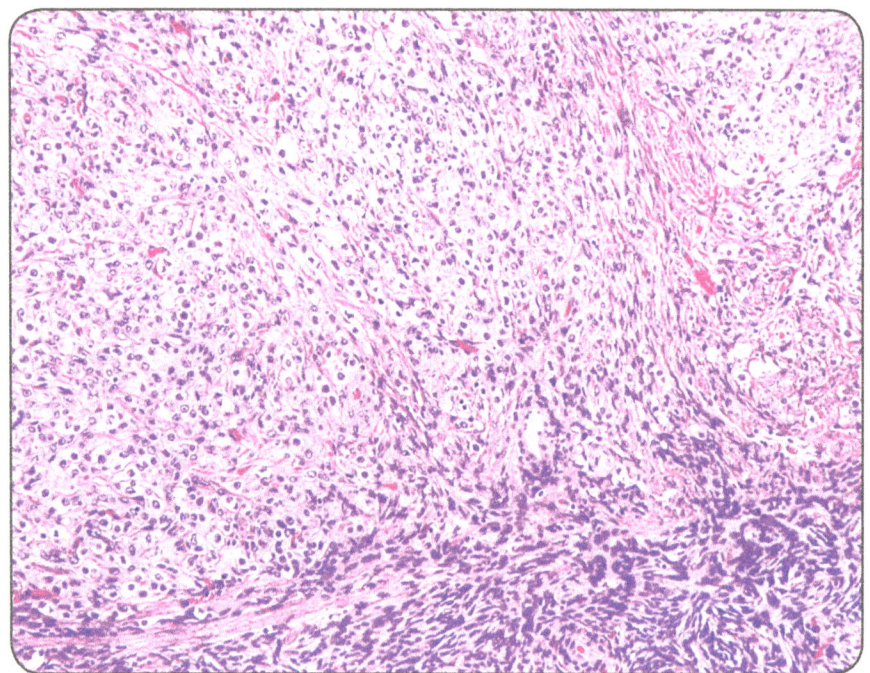

Figure 4.24

Answer: B. Thecoma

Comment: This spindle cell tumor reacts with **Oil-red O** demonstrating an abundance of lipid in tumor cells. In comparison with the normal cortical stromal cells (seen along the lower edge of the Figure 4.24), tumor cells have more abundant clear, lightly eosinophilic cytoplasm, which is typical of **thecoma.** Such luteinization occurs commonly in thecomas and should not be included in the diagnosis. The term **luteinized thecoma** is used for a rare, unique form of thecoma, which shows similar changes but is typically associated with sclerosing peritonitis.

Q.78 Thecomas react with antibodies to all the following antigens, *except:*

  A. CD56
  B. α-inhibin
  C. Calretinin
  D. WT1
  E. CD10

Answer: E. CD10

Comment: **Thecoma** cells react with antibodies that recognize sex-cord stromal cells, such as WT1, CD56, inhibin, but do not react with the antibody to CD10, which may be used as a marker for endometrial stromal cells. Thecomas share some common immunophenotypic features with ovarian fibromas and leiomyomas in that all these tumors are positive for CD56, WT1, estrogen and progesterone receptors (*Source:* He H, et al. Am J Surg Pathol. 2008; 32:884-90).

Q.79 Which ovarian tumor is typically found in patients who have Meigs or Gorlin syndrome?

A. Fibroma
B. Thecoma
C. Adult granulosa cell tumor
D. Endometrial stromal sarcoma
E. Sertoli-Leydig cell tumor

Answer: A. Fibroma

Comment: **Meigs syndrome** includes pleural effusion and ovarian fibroma. **Gorlin syndrome,** also known as nevoid basal cell carcinoma syndrome is characterized by multiple basal cell carcinomas of the skin, odontogenic keratocyst of the jaws, bone malformations, bilateral fibromas of the ovaries or fibromas of the heart. It is a rare disease (1:100,000), related to the mutations of the *PTCH* (patched) gene. The mutation is inherited as an autosomal dominant trait.

Q.80 Which of the following sex cord-stromal tumors occurs predominantly in young women under the age of 30 years?

A. Fibroma
B. Fibrothecoma
C. Thecoma
D. Fibrosarcoma
E. Sclerosing stromal tumor

Answer: E. Sclerosing stromal tumor

Comment: The vast majority of **sclerosing stromal tumors** are found in women under the age of 30 years. Other tumors listed here occur most often in older women with a peak in the 50–60 years age group.

Q.81 What is the best diagnosis for this ovarian tumor from a 28-year-old woman (Figure 4.25)?

A. Fibroma
B. Fibrothecoma
C. Thecoma
D. Fibrosarcoma
E. Sclerosing stromal tumor

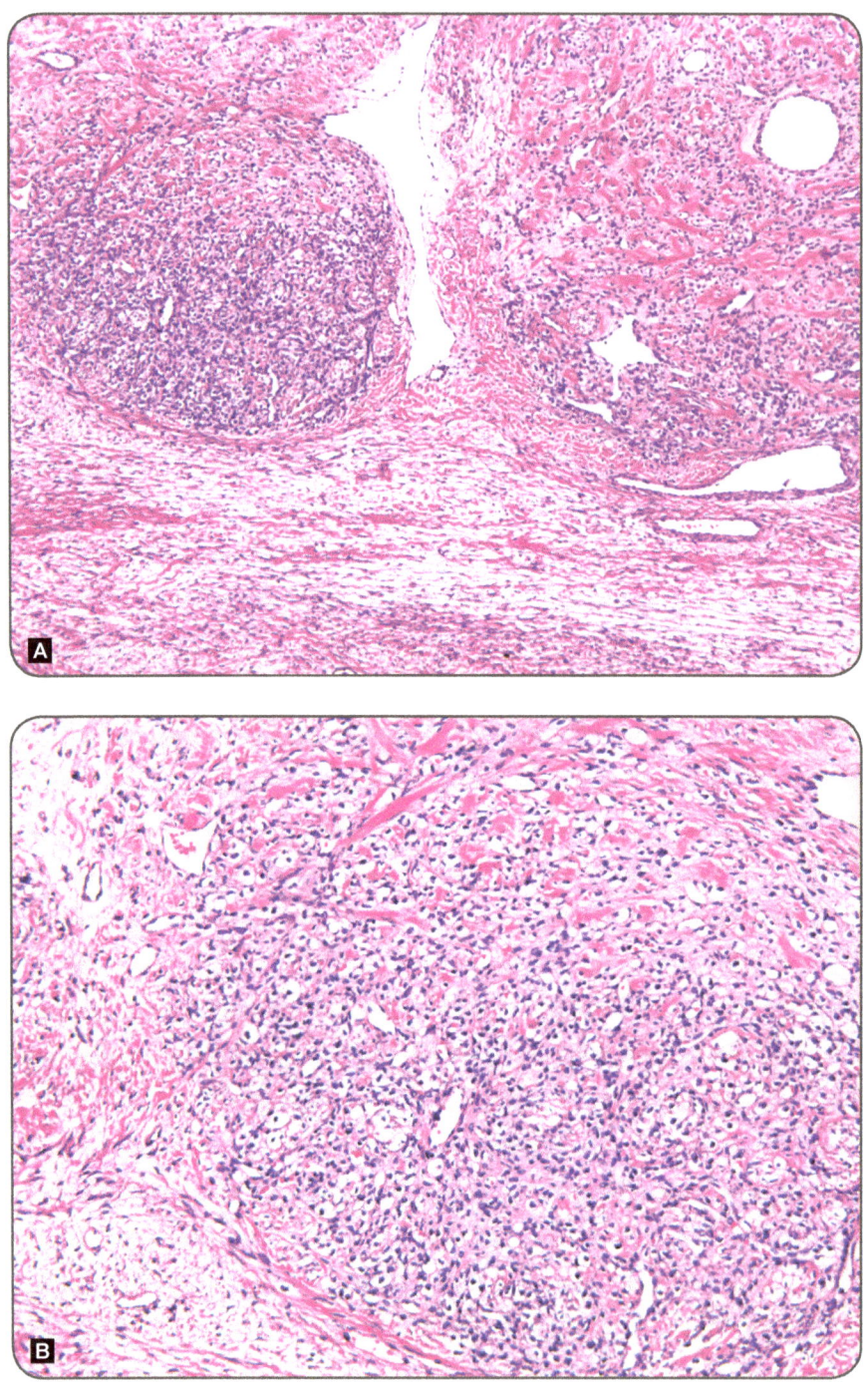

Figures 4.25A and B

Answer: E. Sclerosing stromal tumor

Comment: Figure 4.25 shows the typical features of a **sclerosing stromal tumor** composed of spindle cell nodules separated one from another and the normal ovarian stroma (seen along the lower edge of Figure 4.25A) by loosely structured edematous fibrous tissue. Inside the nodules there are fibroblast-like cells and vacuolated or clear luteinized cells, adjacent to numerous branching thin-walled blood vessels (Figure 4.25B). Sclerosing stromal tumors are benign and usually do not secrete hormones.

Q.82 Microscopic subtyping or grading of which sex cord-stromal ovarian tumor is clinically important for formulating the prognosis of these tumors?

   A. Fibroma
   B. Steroid cell tumor
   C. Thecoma
   D. Sertoli-Leydig cell tumor
   E. Sclerosing stromal tumor

Answer: D. Sertoli-Leydig cell tumor

Comment: Several microscopic variants of Sertoli-Leydig cell tumors (SLCT) are recognized, including the following:
- Well-differentiated SLCT
- SLCT of intermediate differentiation
- Poorly differentiated ("sarcomatoid") SLCT
- Retiform SLCT

Although most SLCT are benign, some poorly differentiated ("sarcomatoid" SLCT) may metastasize. Accordingly, it is essential to classify the tumor and include the subtype of SLCT in the final pathologic diagnosis. Well-differentiated SLCT are invariably benign, but they are the least common subtype. They do not contain heterologous elements, which occur however in a significant number of retiform and intermediate and poorly differentiated tumors. This group of SLCT may also contain neuroendocrine elements, usually in a well-differentiated form (i.e. as carcinoids).

Q.83 What is the most likely diagnostic subtype of this Sertoli-Leydig cell tumor (Figure 4.26)?

   A. Well-differentiated SLCT
   B. SLCT of intermediate differentiation
   C. Poorly differentiated SLCT
   D. Retiform SLCT
   E. SLCT of intermediate differentiation with intestinal heterologous elements

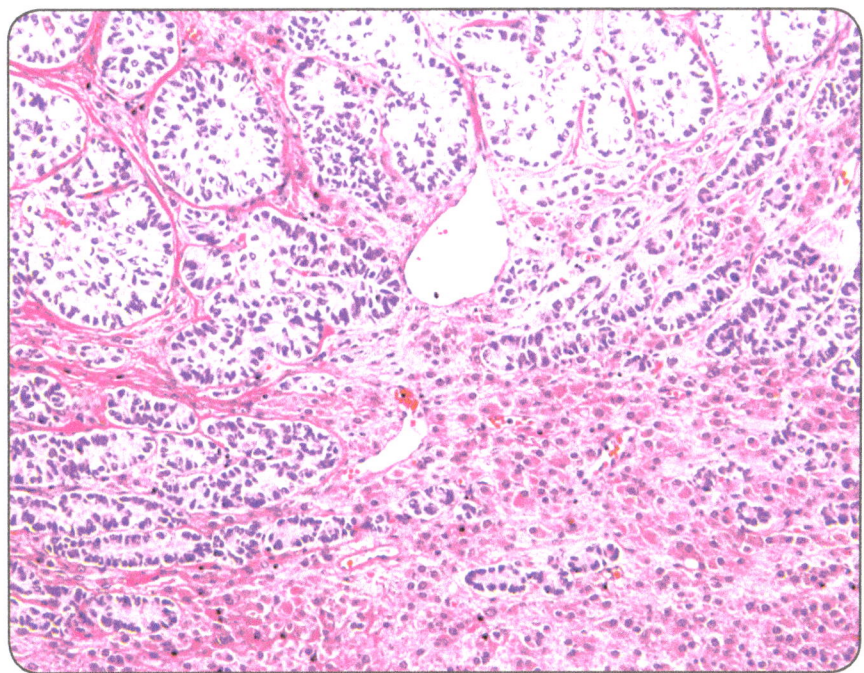

Figure 4.26

Answer: A. Well-differentiated SLCT

Comment: This Sertoli-Leydig cell tumor contains tubules lined by Sertoli-like cells (upper part of the Figure) and nests of cells with eosinophilic cytoplasm resembling Leydig cells (lower part of the Figure), and is thus classified as a well-differentiated SLCT.

Q.84 What is the most likely subtype diagnosis for this SLCT (Figure 4.27)?

- A. Well-differentiated SLCT
- B. SLCT of intermediate differentiation
- C. SLCT of intermediate differentiation with heterologous elements
- D. Poorly differentiated SLCT
- E. Retiform SLCT

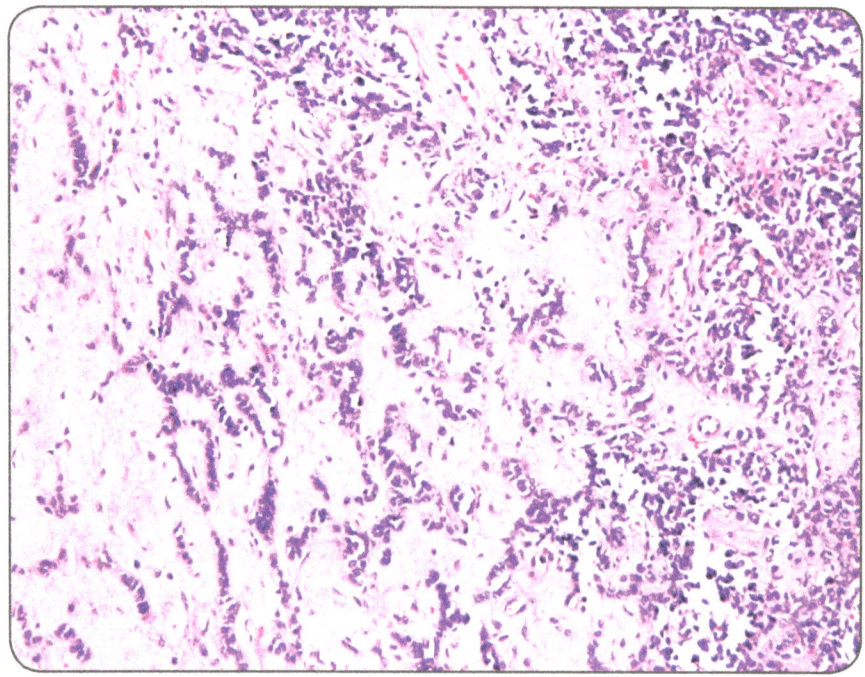

Figure 4.27

Answer: E. Retiform SLCT

Comment: **Retiform SLCT** shown in Figure 4.27 consists of small cuboidal and flattened cells lining inter anastomosing narrow channels, which resemble rete testis.

Q.85 What is the most likely diagnosis for this ovarian tumor removed from a patient with Peutz-Jeghers syndrome (Figure 4.28)?

- A. Adult granulosa cell tumors
- B. Juvenile granulosa cell tumor
- C. Sex cord tumor with annular tubules
- D. Sertoli-Leydig cell tumor
- E. Sclerosing stromal tumor

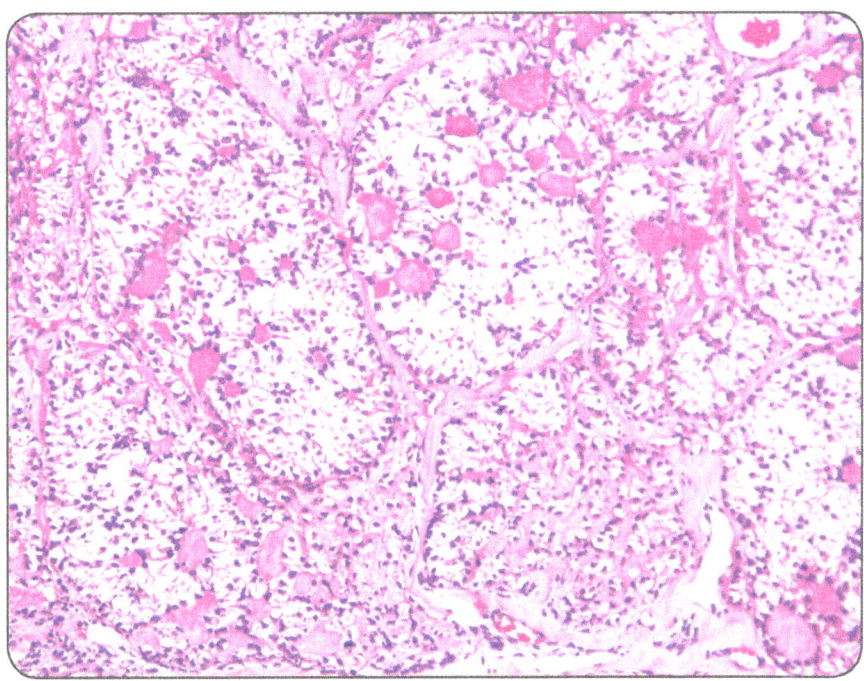

Figure 4.28

Answer: **C. Sex cord tumor with annular tubules**

Comment: This **sex cord tumor with annular tubules** (SCTAT) has unique microscopic features including hyaline bodies surrounded radially with cells that have basally located oval nuclei. In one-third of cases SCTAT are associated with **Peutz-Jeghers syndrome**. Syndromic SCAT may be multiple and are invariably benign, in contrast to sporadic tumors of this kind which may be malignant.

Q.86 All the following are true about steroid tumors of the ovary, *except:*
- **A.** Tumor presents as a solitary mass 5–10 cm in diameter which on cross-section may appear yellow, orange, red or brown
- **B.** Diffuse pattern of cell growth predominates, but cells also may form cords or nests
- **C.** Tumor cells may be lipid rich (clear) or lipid poor (eosinophilic)
- **D.** Androgenic symptoms found in 50% patients
- **E.** Almost invariably benign

Answer: **E. Almost invariably benign**

Comment: **Steroid tumors** are composed of polygonal cells which often but not always contain lipids, and are thus classified as lipid rich or lipid poor. The color of the tumor varies on cross-sections depending on the amount of lipids inside the tumor cells. One-half of tumors cause virilization, but some tumors may secrete estrogens or be hormonally inactive. **Approximately 30% of these tumors are malignant.**

Q.87 All the following are typical pathologic features of Leydig cell tumors of the ovary, *except:*
- **A.** Spindle cells with scant clear lipid rich cytoplasm
- **B.** Clustering of nuclei, leaving fields of nuclear free cytoplasmic
- **C.** Reinke crystals in tumor cell cytoplasm
- **D.** Hilar location
- **E.** Fibrinoid necrosis of blood vessels

Answer: A. Spindle cells with scant clear lipid rich cytoplasm

Comment: **Leydig cell tumors** may contain lipids but in most instances the cells of these tumors have eosinophilic rather than clear cytoplasm. Due to the typical clustering of their nuclei, these tumors usually contain parts composed of eosinophilic cytoplasm free of nuclei. Fibrinoid necrosis and Reinke crystals are additional microscopic features of these tumors which are most often located in the hilum of the ovary.

Q.88 Figure 4.29 shows the microscopic features of a solid ovarian tumor, which was removed from the ovary of a 20-year-old woman. What is the most appropriate diagnosis?

- A. Dysgerminoma
- B. Mixed germ cell tumor
- C. Yolk sac tumor
- D. Carcinoma arising in a teratoma
- E. Choriocarcinoma

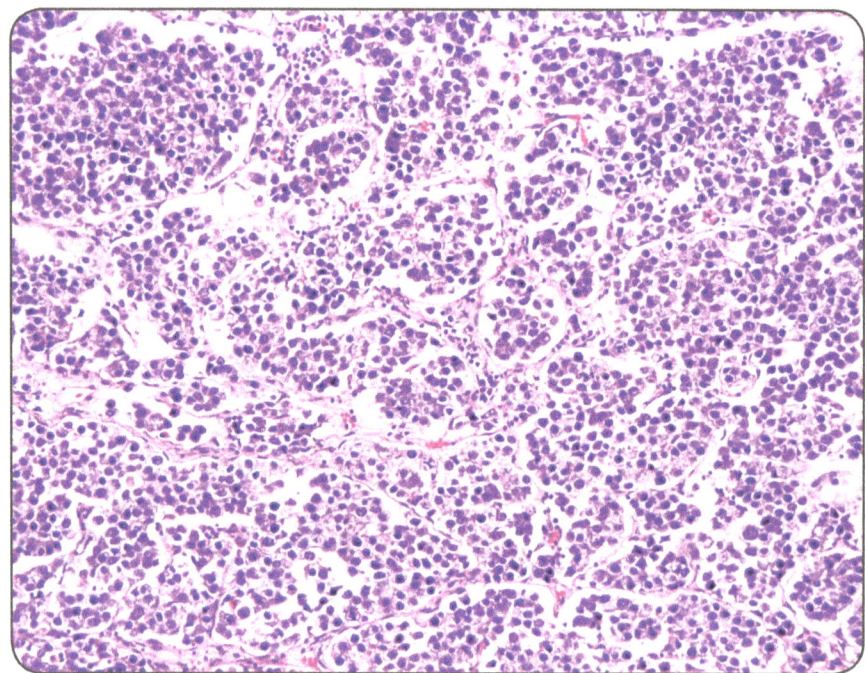

Figure 4.29

Answer: A. Dysgerminoma

Comment: **Dysgerminoma** shown in Figure 4.29 is a germ cell tumor composed of polygonal cells with vesicular nuclei and clear cytoplasm, which is rich in glycogen. Tumor cells are arranged into nests surrounded by fibrous septa infiltrated with lymphocytes.

Q.89 Which one of the following is the most common solid malignant germ cell tumor of the ovary of women under the age of 30 years?

- A. Dysgerminoma
- B. Mixed germ cell tumor
- C. Yolk sac tumor
- D. Carcinoma arising in a teratoma
- E. Choriocarcinoma

Answer: A. Dysgerminoma

Comment: **Dysgerminoma** is the most common malignant germ cell tumor in women under the age of 30 years. Note that this question did not include immature teratomas, which are reported in some papers and textbooks as the most common malignant germ cell tumor in that age group. Furthermore immature teratomas often contain cystic parts. These "nitpicking" details aside, there are no doubts that dysgerminoma and immature teratomas are two most common malignant ovarian germ cell tumors in women under the age of 30 years.

Q.90 Antibodies to which antigen react with the nuclei of dysgerminoma?
- A. Placental alkaline phosphatase (PLAP)
- B. c-KIT (CD117)
- C. Podoplanin (D2-40)
- D. Transcription factor OCT-4
- E. Cytokeratin CK7

Answer: D. Transcription factor OCT-4

Comment: Antibodies to OCT-4 react with nuclei of dysgerminoma and embryonal carcinoma. Antibodies to placental alkaline phosphatase react with the cell membrane and cytoplasm of dysgerminoma cells, whereas antibodies to podoplanin and c-KIT react with the cell membrane of these tumors. Antibodies to cytokeratin CK may react focally in a dot-like manner with the perinuclear cytoplasm or not at all.

Q.91 Antibody to which antigen reacts with the nuclei of all malignant germ cell tumors?
- A. OCT-4
- B. D2-40
- C. CD30
- D. SALL4
- E. Placental alkaline phosphatase (PLAP)

Answer: D. SALL4

Comment: SALL4 (sal-like protein 4) is a gene encoding a transcription factor that has homeotic function during development. It is expressed in the nuclei of essentially all human ovarian and testicular malignant germ cell tumors. Of all other antigens listed here, OCT-4 is the only one also expressed in the nuclei. However, it is expressed only in dysgerminoma, embryonal carcinoma and gonadoblastoma, and does not react with cells of the yolk sac tumor.

Q.92 What is the most common and/or predominant microscopic growth pattern seen in yolk sac carcinoma?
- A. Papillary
- B. Polyvesicular vitelline
- C. Reticular
- D. Hepatoid
- E. Glandular

Answer: C. Reticular

Comment: Most yolk sac carcinomas have several microscopic growth patterns. Reticular, the most common pattern is characterized by the formation of anastomosing channels focally expanding into cystic spaces, all of which are lined cuboidal or flattened cells bordering on loose myxoid stroma.

Q.93 What is the most likely diagnosis for this ovarian tumor removed from a 15-year-old girl (Figure 4.30)?

- A. Dysgerminoma
- B. Mixed germ cell tumor
- C. Yolk sac tumor
- D. Carcinoma arising in a teratoma
- E. Choriocarcinoma

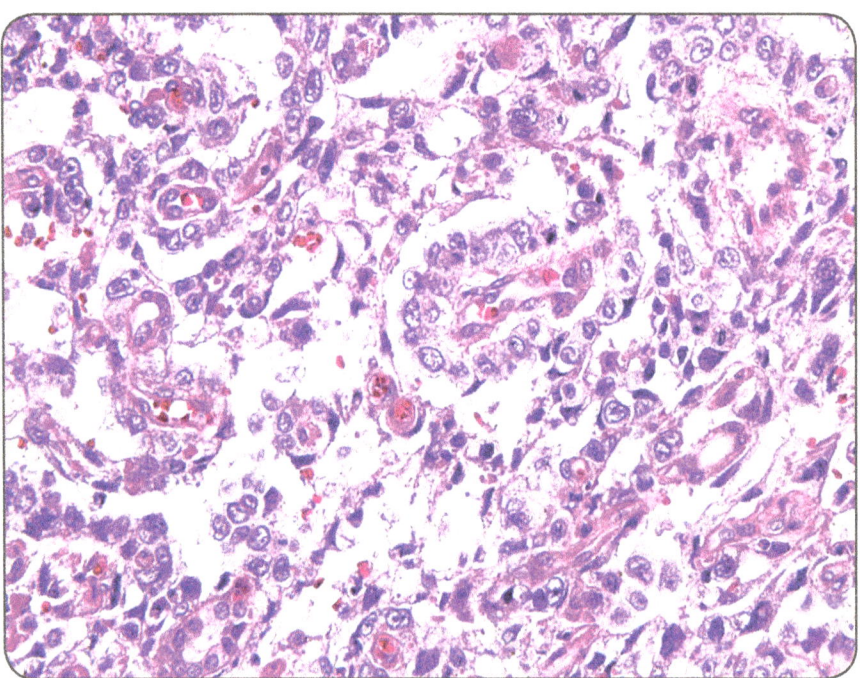

Figure 4.30

Answer: **C. Yolk sac tumor**

Comment: Figure 4.30 shows several patterns, although the reticular pattern predominates. Several growth patterns intermixed one with another are the hallmark of yolk sac tumors. The variegated appearance of the tumor is the basic clue to the diagnosis even if the supposedly diagnostic glomeruloid Schiller-Duval bodies are not found.

Q.94 Which of the following is the best serum marker for the laboratory diagnosis of yolk sac carcinoma of the ovary?

- A. Alpha fetoprotein
- B. Lactic dehydrogenase
- C. Placental alkaline phosphatase
- D. CA125
- E. Neuron-specific enolase

Answer: **A. Alpha fetoprotein**

Comment: **Alpha fetoprotein** (AFP) is a normal fetal serum glycoprotein produced by yolk sac cells and the fetal liver. Concentrations of AFP in serum drop gradually and reach normal levels by the end of the first postnatal year. High serum concentration of AFP, usually above 1,000 ng/mL, are found in all patients with yolk sac tumors. Following the tumor resection serum concentration of AFP will gradually decrease, depending on the completeness of the tumor surgery. The actual half-life of serum AFP following the resection of an AFP secreting tumor is 4–6 days. Hence, AFP is also a useful serologic marker for the follow-up of treated patients.

Q.95 Glypican-3 is a good tumor marker for which tumor of the ovary?

    A. Dysgerminoma
    B. High-grade serous carcinoma
    C. Yolk sac tumor
    D. Immature teratoma
    E. Clear cell carcinoma

Answer: **C. Yolk sac carcinoma**

Comment: **Glypican-3** is a useful, albeit not entirely specific marker for yolk sac tumor. It is not expressed in dysgerminoma, but may be found focally in some teratomas. It is not found in serous and mucinous and most clear cell carcinomas of the ovary. However, it may be also expressed in some clear cells carcinomas of the ovary (*Source:* Esheba GE, et al. Am J Surg Pathol. 2008;32: 600-7).

Q.96 Which immature tissue is most important for the pathologic evaluation of immature teratomas?

    A. Fetal neuroectodermal tubules and rosettes
    B. Embryonal intestines
    C. Fetal liver
    D. Fetal kidney
    E. Fetal pancreas

Answer: **A. Fetal neuroectodermal tubules and rosettes**

Comment: **Immature neural tissue**, which most often presents in form of fetal neuroectodermal tubules and rosettes is the most common immature component of **immature teratomas**. The extent of immature neural tissues is used quantitatively to divide immature teratomas into two groups: High-grade and low-grade tumors.

Q.97 Which one of the following is the most common germ cell tumor of the ovary?

    A. Cystic teratoma
    B. Solid teratoma
    C. Immature teratoma with neural rosettes
    D. Immature teratoma with embryoid bodies
    E. Mixed germ cell tumor-like

Answer: **A. Cystic teratoma**

Comment: **Cystic teratomas** account for more than 90% of all ovarian germ cell tumors. These tumors originate from parthenogenetically activated germ cells. They can be diagnosed in any age group, but usually in the first half of the reproductive period.

Q.98 Which tissue is most often found in cystic ovarian teratomas?

    A. Skin
    B. Neural tissue
    C. Bone
    D. Cartilage
    E. Dental tissue

Answer: A. Skin

Comment: **Ectodermal tissues** predominate in **cystic ovarian teratomas**. Among these, skin is the most predominant element. Hence, the widely used synonym **dermoid cyst**.

Q.99 Which ovarian tumor represents the most common monodermal teratoma?
- A. Carcinoid
- B. Struma ovarii
- C. Ependymoma
- D. Neuroectodermal carcinoma
- E. Astrocytoma

Answer: B. Struma ovarii

Comment: **Monodermal teratomas** are tumors composed of a single somatic tissue. **Struma ovarii** composed microscopically of thyroid tissue is the most common monodermal teratoma.

Thyroid tissue is a common component of cystic teratomas and it is found in approximately 20% benign teratomas. Tumors composed exclusively or predominantly of thyroid tissue, i.e. **strumae ovarii** are approximately ten times less common.

Q.100 Figure 4.31 shows two somatic tissue in a cystic teratoma. What are they?
- A. Cartilage and bone
- B. Bone and squamous epithelium
- C. Squamous epithelium and cartilage
- D. Cartilage and skeletal muscle
- E. Neural tissue and bone

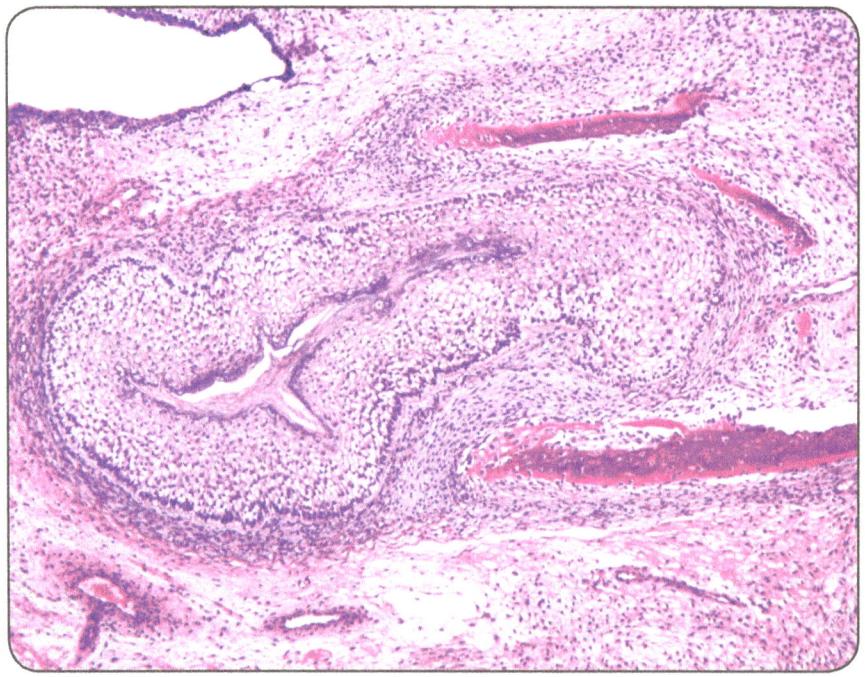

Figure 4.31

Answer: B. Bone and squamous epithelium

Comment: On the right side of the Figure 4.31 one may see three eosinophilic spicules of bone, enclosing an oval structure composed of squamous epithelium. Note that the fetal squamous epithelium is glycogen rich, and the cells thus have a clear cytoplasm.

Q.101 Figure 4.32 shows a germ cell tumor. What is the most likely diagnosis?
- A. Cystic teratoma, mature
- B. Immature teratoma
- C. Carcinoma arising in a benign teratoma
- D. Yolk sac tumor and teratoma
- E. Embryonal carcinoma in a teratoma

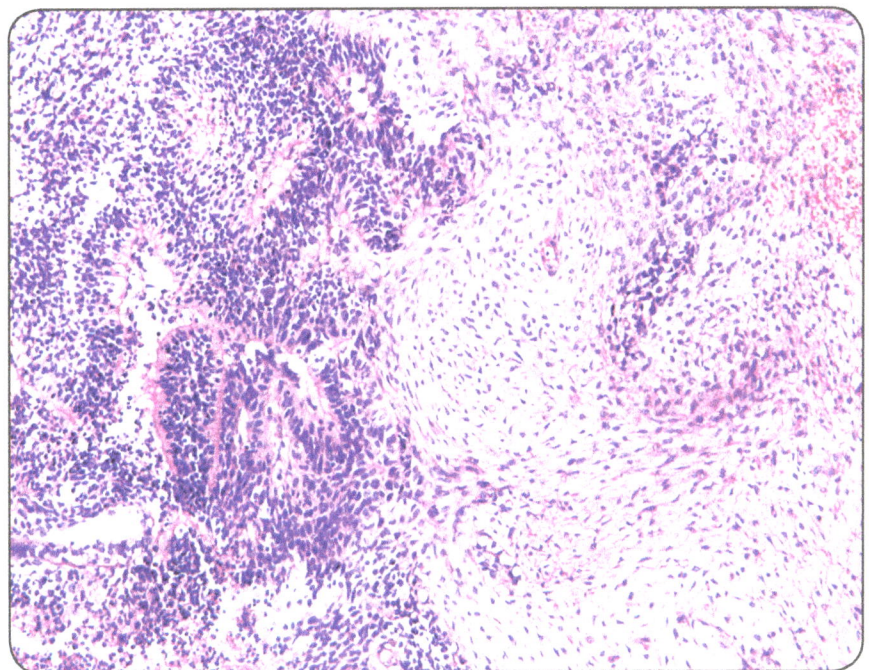

Figure 4.32

Answer: B. Immature teratoma

Comment: The left side of the Figure 4.32 shows immature neural cells, partially arranged into neural tubes. These immature neural cells are typical features of **immature teratoma**.

Q.102 What is the most likely diagnosis for this tumor identified as a small nodule in a cystic teratoma (Figure 4.33)?
- A. Adenocarcinoma
- B. Squamous cell carcinoma
- C. Carcinoid
- D. Malignant melanoma
- E. Lymphoma

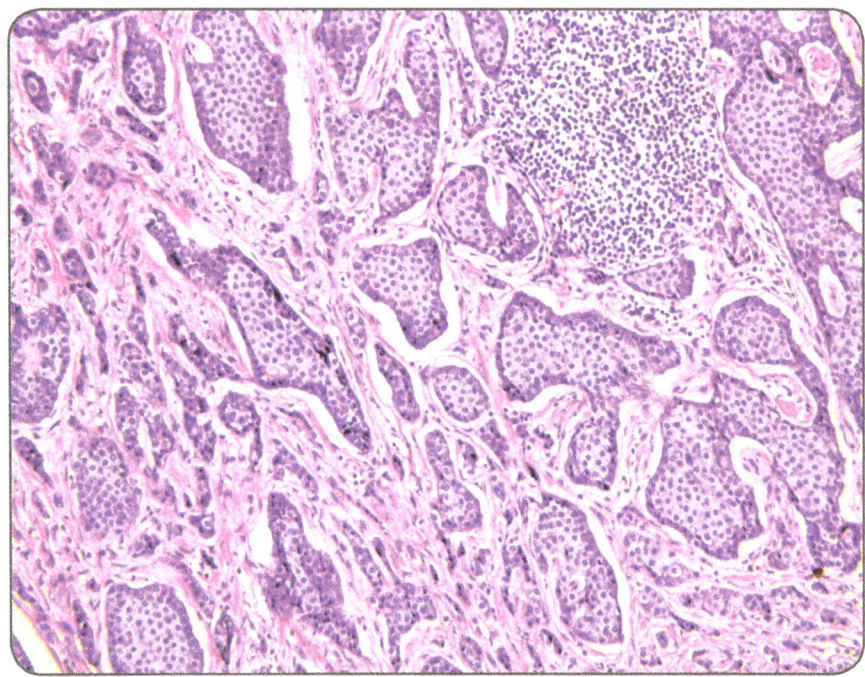

Figure 4.33

Answer: C. Carcinoid

Comment: Like this tumor (Figure 4.33), most **carcinoids** of the ovary have an insular architecture and are low-grade malignant tumors. Less often they are trabecullar or mucinous. Most of these carcinoids are small and innocuous.

Q.103 What is the most common endocrine/neuroendocrine tumor originating in ovarian teratomas?

    A. Papillary carcinoma of the thyroid
    B. Follicular carcinoma of the thyroid
    C. Medullary carcinoma of the thyroid
    D. Undifferentiated carcinoma of the thyroid
    E. Carcinoid

Answer: E. Carcinoid

Comment: Ovarian **carcinoids** (neuroendocrine tumors grade I) are rare and yet they are the most common neuroendocrine tumors originating in teratomas of the ovary. In addition to carcinoids in teratomas, there are carcinoids originating within a struma ovarii. Isolated ovarian carcinoid, apparently unrelated to teratoma or any other tumor, and thus representing true monodermal teratomas, are also on record. Overall, ovarian carcinoids account for less than 1% of all carcinoids, and for 0.1% of all ovarian tumors. Carcinoid syndrome is present in patients with larger tumors, and most of those that were analyzed were classified microscopically as insular carcinoids.

Q.104 Figure 4.34 shows a malignant tumor originating in a benign cystic teratoma of 60-year-old woman? What is the most likely diagnosis?

    A. Adenocarcinoma
    B. Squamous cell carcinoma
    C. Small cell carcinoma
    D. Malignant melanoma
    E. Lymphoma

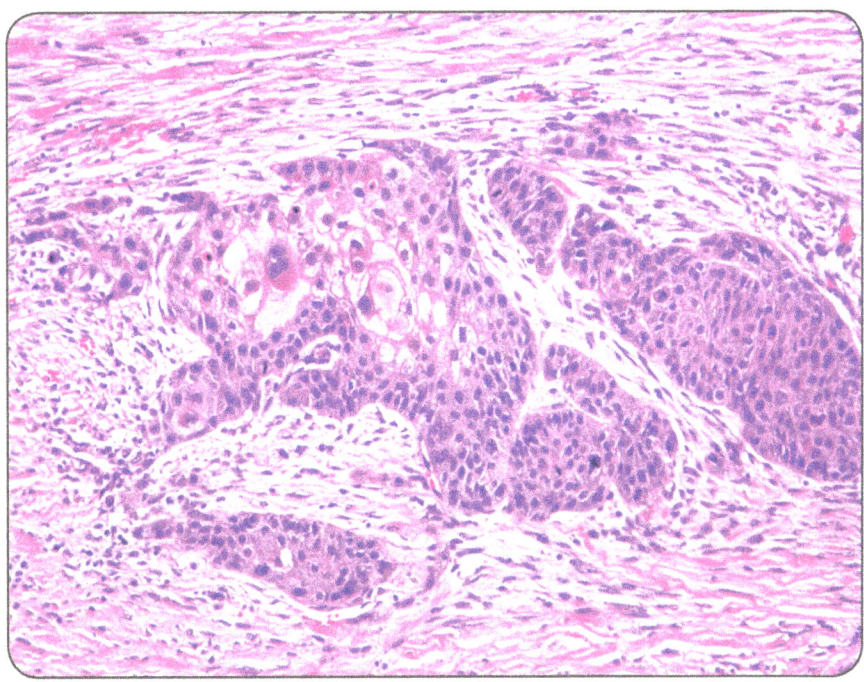

Figure 4.34

Answer: **B. Squamous cell carcinomas**

Comment: The tumor shown in Figure 4.34 is a **squamous cell carcinoma** composed of irregular nests of atypical cells, some extending into invasive strands and minimal keratinization.

Q.105 **What is the most common secondary malignancy arising in cystic teratomas of the ovary?**

A. Adenocarcinoma
B. Squamous cell carcinoma
C. Sarcoma
D. Malignant melanoma
E. Lymphoma

Answer: **B. Squamous cell carcinoma**

Comment: **Squamous cell carcinomas** are the most common malignant tumors originating in cystic teratomas. These tumors account for 80% of all secondary malignancies in cystic teratomas. Adenocarcinomas, which are the second most common malignancy in teratomas, are ten times less common. Sarcomas originating in cystic teratomas are rare.

Q.106 **What is the most common malignant invasive tumor originating in gonadoblastomas?**

A. Gonocytoma
B. Yolk sac tumor
C. Embryonal carcinoma
D. Mixed germ cell tumor
E. Sertoli cell tumor

Answer: **A. Gonocytoma**

Comment: Most tumors originating in **gonadoblastomas** have the same microscopic features as ovarian dysgerminomas or testicular seminomas. However, since most of these malignancies arise in indeterminate gonads of phenotypic females who have a Y chromosome, it is best to use a non-committal term and call them **gonocytoma**.

Q.107 Figure 4.35 shows the microscopic features of a tumor involving symmetrically both ovaries in a 54-year-old woman. Each ovary measured 9 cm in largest diameter and had a smooth external surface without obvious nodularity. Tumor cells reacted positively with mucicarmine special stain. What is the most likely diagnosis?

- A. Dysgerminoma
- B. Metastatic carcinoma from the gastrointestinal tract
- C. High-grade serous carcinomas
- D. Low-grade mucinous carcinomas
- E. Goblet cell carcinoid

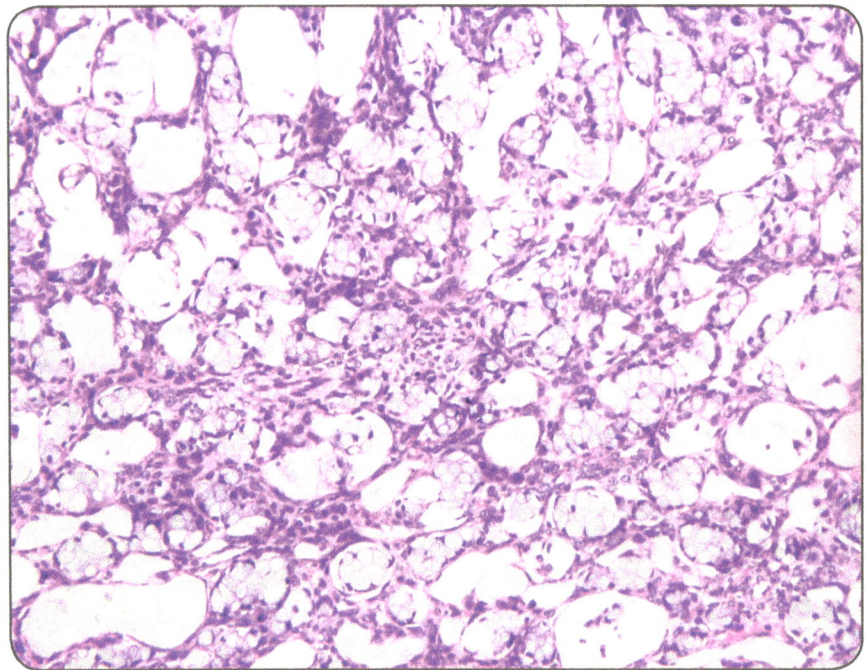

Figure 4.35

Answer: B. Metastatic carcinoma from the gastrointestinal tract

Comment: The tumor shown in Figure 4.34 is an adenocarcinoma. The tumor is composed of mucin rich clear cells forming tightly packed glands with imperceptible lumina. Most tumors of this kind, represent **metastases** from a primary in the gastrointestinal tract. Carcinomas originating from gastric or rectal primaries have a CK7+, CK20- immunophenotype, whereas those of appendiceal and colonic origin are usually CK7-, CK20+. Eponymically they are often called **Krukenberg tumors,** even though they do not have the classical single signet-ring cell appearance originally described by this German author.

CHAPTER 5

Placenta

Q.1 What is the most common uterine site of implantation of the human blastocyst?

   A. Cervical canal
   B. Lower uterine segment
   C. Anterior wall of the endometrial cavity
   D. Posterior wall of endometrial cavity, midportion to upper part
   E. Fundus of the uterus

Answer: D. Posterior wall of endometrial cavity, midportion to upper part

Comment: Most human blastocysts **implant** on the posterior side of the uterus, usually in the midportion or the upper part.

Q.2 Which cells on the implanting conceptus invade the uterine decidua, the myometrium, and the decidual spiral arteries?

   A. Amniotic cells
   B. Chorion laeve
   C. Villi of chorion frondosum
   D. Syncytiotrophoblastic cells
   E. Extravillous cytotrophoblastic cell

Answer: E. Extravillous cytotrophoblastic cells

Comment: Cytotrophoblastic cells detaching from the anchoring villi of the implanting embryo correspond to the **extravillous or intermediate trophoblast**. These cells invade the decidua, the superficial layer of the myometrium, and the decidual spiral arteries. Depending on their location they are called **interstitial** extravillous trophoblast or **intravascular** extravillous trophoblast. These cells can be identified immunohistochemically with antibodies to cytokeratins and human placental lactogen.

Q.3 Indications for the pathologic examination of the placenta are usually classified as maternal, fetal and placental. Which of the following is considered to be a placental indication for the examination of the placenta?

   A. Maternal diabetes mellitus
   B. Preeclampsia
   C. Prematurity
   D. Fetal demise
   E. Amniotic bands

Answer: E. Amniotic bands

Comment: **Amniotic bands** seen by naked eye examination of the placenta belong to **placental indications** for pathologic examination of placentas. Other anatomic abnormalities of the placenta or the umbilical cord noted by the obstetrician also mandate a pathologic examination. Examples of **maternal indications** include maternal diseases known to affect the pregnancy, such as hypertension, diabetes mellitus or preeclampsia. **Fetal indications** include grossly visible developmental abnormalities of the fetus, marked growth retardation or fetus/neonate-related complications of pregnancy and delivery.

Q.4 During the gross examination of the placenta the pathologist noted an incompleteness of the maternal surface. Which of the following placental abnormalities will most likely cause this defect?
   A. Placenta accreta
   B. Placenta praevia
   C. Placenta circumvallata
   D. Placenta circummarginalis
   E. Vellamentous insertion of the cord

Answer: A. Placenta accreta

Comment: **Placenta accreta** may result in the retention of maternal side chorionic villi inside the uterus. Other placental abnormalities listed here do not affect the maternal surface of the placenta.

Q.5 In how many pregnancies (expressed in percentages) does one find a two vessel umbilical cord ("single umbilical artery cord")?
   A. 1%
   B. 5%
   C. 10%
   D. 20%
   E. 30%

Answer: A. 1%

Comment: **Single umbilical artery** is found in somewhat less than 1% of all placentas.

Q.6 What is the outcome of pregnancy associated with two vessel umbilical cords?
   A. Unremarkable—most infants are normal
   B. Trisomy 18 is found in 20% infants
   C. Congenital heart disease is found in 30% infants
   D. Renal malformations are found in 50% infants
   E. Central nervous anomalies are found in 60% infants

Answer: A. Unremarkable—most infants are normal

Comment: Even though most infants born in pregnancies characterized by **two vessel umbilical cord** are normal, there is a slightly **increased incidence** of all those pathological changes listed here. Preterm deliveries and growth restrictions have been reported in some studies. Overall, single artery cord seems to be associated with adverse outcomes, but the true incidence of these cannot be determined.

Q.7 Which form of umbilical cord insertion is most often associated with fetal pathology?

A. Paracentral
B. Central
C. Eccentric
D. Marginal
E. Velamentous

Answer: **E. Velamentous**

Comment: **Velamentous insertion** of the umbilicus is characterized by a lack of Wharton jelly in the cord, rendering the cord more susceptible to compression, rupture or thrombosis with consequent fetal ischemia.

A few words about insertion of the umbilical cord seem to be appropriate here. Paracentral insertion is the most common type of umbilical cord insertion. Central and eccentric insertions are also common and they are inconsequential. Marginal insertion is also innocuous unless associated with velamentous vessels, which are more susceptible to injury and thrombosis.

Q.8 Which form of umbilical cord insertion is most often associated with vasa previa?

A. Paracentral
B. Central
C. Eccentric
D. Marginal
E. Velamentous

Answer: **E. Velamentous**

Comment: In **velamentous insertion,** the umbilical cord vessels usually branch externally to the membranes which also contain prominent vasculature. If such membranes cover the internal cervical os they form so called *vasa previa,* which, due to their location, are prone to injury, bleeding, and thrombosis. Other forms of insertion are not associated with vasa previa. An increased incidence of vasa previa has been reported in multiple gestations and in association with two vessel umbilical cords.

Q.9 The most common umbilical cord inclusions found microscopically are derived from which structure?

A. Allantoic duct
B. Amnion
C. Chorion
D. Yolk sac
E. Omphalomesenteric duct

Answer: **A. Allantoic duct**

Comment: Various **epithelial inclusions** or **cysts** are found in about 20% microscopically examined umbilical cords. The most common are allantoic duct inclusions which present as epithelial nests, ducts or cysts lined by transitional or flattened cuboidal epithelium. Like the foci of squamous metaplasia on the external surface of the umbilical cord, these epithelial inclusions are of no clinical significance. Larger cysts may be detected by ultrasound. Exceptionally rarely, they may become infected.

Q.10 Amnion nodosum is most often found in which condition?

A. Polyhydramnios
B. Oligohydramnios
C. Chorioamnionitis

D. Umbilical pseudonodules
E. Tight umbilical cord nodules

Answer: B. Oligohydramnios

Comment: **Oligohydramnios** leads to focal loss of amniotic epithelium due to a lack of nutrients in scant amniotic fluid. Necrosis of cells results in a defect which is covered with amorphous and lanugo hair from the amniotic fluid. Excessive accumulation of this material results in **amnion nodosum.**

Polyhydramnios does not affect the amniotic epithelium.

Chorioamnionitis presents with typical signs of inflammation, such as a fibrinopurulent exudate or in milder cases grossly visible opacification of membranes.

Umbilical pseudonodules are varicosities of umbilical vessels, and they are of no clinical significance.

Tight true cord nodules may cause fetal ischemia and are associated with increased fetal mortality, estimated to be around 10%.

Q.11 Acute chorioamnionitis is found most often in the placenta delivered spontaneously at which week of pregnancy?

A. 21 week
B. 28 week
C. 32 week
D. 35 week
E. 39 week

Answer: A. 21 week

Comment: Microscopic evidence of chorioamnionitis is inversely proportional to the duration of pregnancy. It is found in over 90% of placentae delivered at 21–24 weeks and only in 3-5% in term pregnancies (*Source:* Kim CJ, et al. Am J Obstet Gynecol. 2015; 213 (suppl 4): S29-S52).

Q.12 What is the most common cause of infectious acute chorioamnionitis?

A. Bacteria
B. Viruses
C. Parasites
D. Fungi
E. Nematodes

Answer: A. Bacteria

Comment: Bacterial infections occur most often by the ascending route through the cervix. Microbiological isolates most often contain Streptococci, uropathogens or *Ureaplasma sp.* In about one-third of microscopically documented cases of acute chorioamnionitis no bacterial pathogens can be demonstrated (*Source:* Romero R, et al. J Perinat Med. 2015; 43:19-36). Chorioamnionitis is a common cause of premature rupture of fetal membranes.

Q.13 Which of the following microscopic findings is typically associated with the most prominent neonatal infection/sepsis?

A. Neutrophils in subchorionic fibrin
B. Neutrophils in chorion and amnion
C. Neutrophils in the wall of umbilical vein
D. Neutrophils in the wall of umbilical artery
E. Necrotizing funisitis

Answer: E. Necrotizing funisitis

Comment: **Necrotizing funisitis**, i.e. purulent inflammation of the umbilical cord with foci of necrosis, is most often associated with prominent neonatal infection/sepsis.

The severity of microscopic chorioamnionitis and funisitis can be estimated (staged from 1 to 3) by taking into consideration the involvement of maternal or fetal structures. Inflammation of chorion and amnion or subchorionic fibrin are signs of **maternal inflammation**, whereas neutrophils in the wall of umbilical veins, arteries or perivascular Wharton jelly are typically associated with **fetal inflammatory response** and/or infection. The staging of the maternal and fetal inflammatory response is given in the Table 5.1.

Both maternal and fetal inflammatory response are graded as severe (grade 2) or not-severe (grade 1).

Table 5.1: Staging of the maternal and fetal inflammatory responses in ascending intrauterine infection, according to the recommendations of the Society of Pediatric Pathology

Maternal inflammatory response	*Fetal inflammatory response*
Stage 1: Acute subchorionitis or chorionitis	Stage 1: Chorionic vasculitis or umbilical phlebitis
Stage 2: Acute chorioamnionitis: polymorphonuclear leukocytes extend into fibrous chorion and/or amnion	Stage 2: Acute umbilical phlebitis and arteritis
Stage 3: Necrotizing chorioamnionitis	Stage 3: Necrotizing funisitis involving the perivascular parts of the umbilicus

Source: Redline RW, et al. Pediatr Dev Pathol. 2003;6:435-48; Khong TY, et al. Arch Pathol Lab Med. 2016;140:698-713.

Q.14 Figure 5.1 shows microscopic changes in a term placenta. These changes are most often associated with which other placental lesion?

A. Acute deciduitis
B. Acute chorioamnionitis
C. Villitis of unknown etiology
D. Thrombosis of placental veins
E. Maternal systemic lupus erythematosus

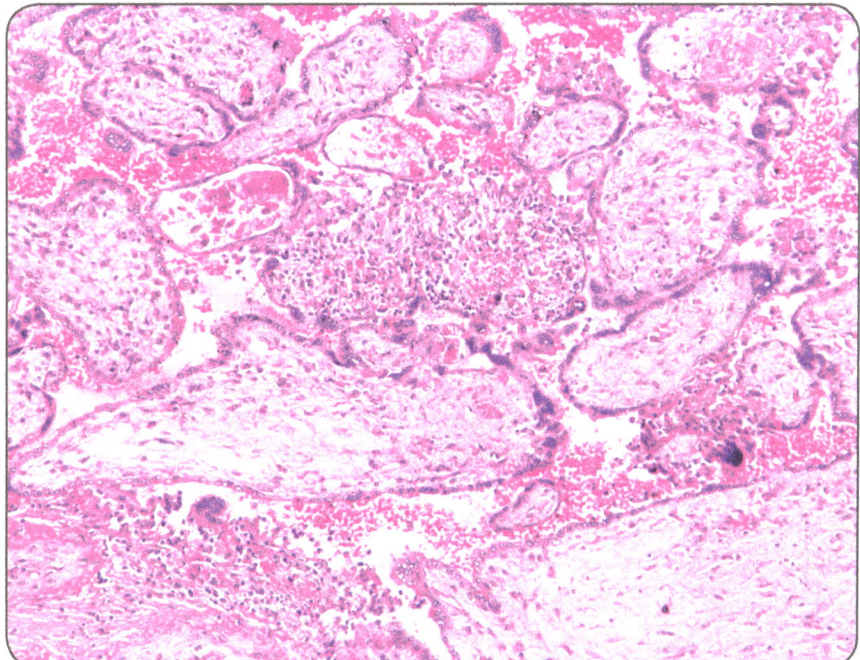

Figure 5.1

Answer: C. Villitis of unknown etiology

Comment: Figure 5.1 shows chronic intervillositis. **Chronic intervillositis, eosinophilic/T-cell vasculitis,** and **chronic deciduitis** are most often associated with **villitis of unknown etiology** (VUE). The etiology and the clinical significance of all these placental lesions is not fully understood.

Chronic villitis of unknown etiology may be graded as mild or severe, which is of clinical significance. Severe VUE is significantly more often associated with fetal growth retardation, neurodevelopmental impairment, and likelihood of recurrence in subsequent pregnancies than mild VUE (*Source:* Khong TY, et al. Arch Pathol Lab Med. 2016;140: 698-713).

Q.15 Which of the following placental pathologic changes is diagnostic of human immunodeficiency virus infection?

    A. Obliterative endarteritis
    B. Lymphocytic-plasmacytic villitis
    C. Villous capillary thrombosis
    D. Multinucleated giant cells
    E. None of the above

Answer: E. None of the above

Comment: There are no placental histopathologic changes that are diagnostic of **HIV infection.** Obliterative endarteritis may be seen in syphilis, and it may be combined with lymphocytic-plasmacytic villitis. However, chronic inflammation may be seen in other infections, such as cytomegalovirus (CMV) infection, which can be recognized by the presence of intranuclear inclusions in enlarged cells. Thrombi in the villous capillaries and hemosiderin deposition are also seen in CMV infection. Multinucleated giant cells are prominent in some viral diseases, such as *varicella-zoster* infection.

Q.16 Which pathogen typically causes acute villitis and intervillous abscesses?

    A. *Treponema pallidum*
    B. *Toxoplasma gondii*
    C. Parvovirus B19
    D. *Listeria monocytogenes*
    E. Herpes simplex virus type 2

Answer: D. *Listeria monocytogenes*

Comment: **Listeria monocytogenes** infection of the placenta is characterized by infiltrates of neutrophils in the chorionic villi and intervillous abscesses.

Treponema pallidum presents with lymphocytic-plasma cellular villitis and obliterative vasculitis.

Toxoplasma gondii causes chronic villitis with focal calcification.

Parvovirus B19 infection is associated with villitis and intervillitis and nucleated red blood cells in the villous capillaries. Some RBC show central nuclear clearing with margination of chromatin. Virus is best demonstrated by immunohistochemistry.

Herpes simplex virus (HSV) infection in the first trimester may infect placenta and cause plasma cell rich villitis with hemosiderin deposits. One may see multinucleated giant cell change in decidua and intervillous trophoblast. HSV as well as cytomegalovirus (CMV) are best demonstrated in microscopic slides by immunohistochemical stains.

Q.17 Meconium in amniotic fluid is taken up in macrophages in various parts of the placenta, cord, and fetal membranes. Approximately, 1 hour after the discharge of the meconium from the infants intestines the pigment is first seen in macrophages in which location?

A. Amnion
B. Chorion
C. Decidua
D. Wharton jelly of the umbilicus
E. Umbilical vessels

Answer: **A. Amnion**

Comment: Brown **meconium** pigment is first seen in macrophages of the amnion at about 1 hour from the discharge of fetal intestinal contents. Thereafter, it appears in macrophages of the chorion (at 3 hours), and a few hours later in macrophages in other anatomic sites. Meconium also affects the amniotic epithelium on the fetal surface of the placental disc. These cells become tall cuboidal, vacuolated and tend to pile up.

Q.18 In which of the following maternal/fetal disorders is the placenta usually larger than normal?

A. Down syndrome
B. Intrauterine fetal growth retardation
C. Anencephaly
D. Maternal preeclampsia
E. Maternal diabetes mellitus

Answer: **E. Maternal diabetes mellitus**

Comment: Infants born to **diabetic women** tend to weigh more than others, and also have a larger placenta. In contrast to them, preeclampsia is usually associated with reduced placental weight. Intrauterine fetal growth retardation, malformations involving major organ system, and chromosomal abnormalities are associated with smaller than normal placentas.

Q.19 Chorionic villi may invade the myometrium and penetrate all the way to the peritoneal covering of the myometrium. Which of the following placental abnormalities is characterized by such invasion?

A. Placenta accreta
B. Placenta increta
C. Placenta percreta
D. Placenta succenturiata
E. Placenta fenestrata

Answer: **C. Placenta percreta**

Comment: **Placenta percreta** is characterized by the penetration of the chorionic villi throughout the entire thickness of the myometrium all the way to the peritoneum.
Placenta accreta is adherent to the myometrium due to absence or underdevelopment of decidua.
Placenta increta involves invasion of myometrium but to a lesser extent than in placenta percreta.
In **placenta succenturiata** and **placenta fenestrata** there is no myometrial invasion. **Placenta succenturiata** is characterized by an accessory lobe. In **placenta fenestrata,** there are membrane-replaced parenchymal defects in the body of the placental disc and thus the placenta appears fenestrated.

Q.20 What is the name for the abnormally thin placenta covering evenly the entire surface of the uterine cavity?

A. Placenta circumvallata
B. Battledore placenta
C. Placenta praevia
D. Placenta membranacea
E. Bilobed placenta

Answer: D. Placenta membranacea

Comment: Placenta covering evenly the entire surface of the uterine cavity in form of a thin layer is called **placenta membranacea**.

Battledore placenta is another name for the placenta with marginal insertion of the cord. It was named after the badminton racket which has a small head attached to a thin handle.

Placenta circumvallata is encircled with a ring-like raised border attached to membranes doubled back over its edges.

Placenta praevia covers partially or completely the internal os of the endocervical canal.

Bilobed placenta consists of two separate parts separated one from another by membranes.

Q.21 Atherosis of decidual spiral arteries is a sign of which pregnancy problem?

- A. Hypoperfusion of the placenta
- B. Polyhydramnios
- C. Oligohydramnios
- D. Abnormal placentation
- E. Abruptio placentae

Answer: A. Hypoperfusion of the placenta

Comment: **Atherosis of decidual spiral arteries** is marked by fibrin deposition in the wall of spiral decidual arteries, accumulation of foamy macrophages in the intima of these vessels, and perivascular infiltrates of lymphocytes. It is characteristic of **maternal hypoperfusion of the placenta**. Most often it is found in women suffering from preeclampsia, but also it may be seen in some forms of congenital thrombophilia, acquired coagulopathies, systemic lupus erythematosus, scleroderma, and even women with diabetes and essential hypertension. Depositions of fibrin in the wall of the damaged arteries, followed by a formation of intravascular thrombi and even rupture of the vessel wall are signs of vascular injury. Characteristic intimal infiltrates of foamy macrophages, which act as scavenger cells, represent a reaction to vascular injury. In 10% of cases, atherosis of spiral arteries of the basal decidua occurs without any obvious causes in healthy women (*Source:* Alneas-Katjavivi P, et al. Placenta. 2016;37:26-33).

Q.22 All the following changes occur more often in preeclampsia than in normal pregnancies, *except:*

- A. Decidual blood vessel thrombi and fibrinoid necrosis
- B. Increased syncytial knots in the chorionic villi
- C. Multiple infarcts of the placenta
- D. Retroplacental hematomas
- E. Polyhydramnios

Answer: E. Polyhydramnios

Comment: **Preeclampsia** is not associated with **polyhydramnios**, and it is actually more likely to present with **oligohydramnios**. Other changes listed here are signs of **placental hypoperfusion** and/or ischemia. The causes of retroplacental hematomas in preeclampsia are not known, but most likely they are related to other uterine vascular changes in this disease.

Q.23 Which of the following clinical findings is a constant feature of HELLP syndrome, a complication of preeclampsia?

- A. Hemolysis
- B. Elevated blood pressure
- C. Low serum albumin
- D. Thrombocytosis
- E. Leukocytosis

Answer: A. Hemolysis

Comment: **HELLP** syndrome includes **hemolysis, elevated liver enzymes, low platelet** count often resulting in subcapsular liver hematoma and even intracerebral hemorrhage. Other signs of preeclampsia are also present. Fetal death may occur and is often preceded by abruption of the placenta.

Q.24 What is the chorionic-amniotic structure of most monozygotic twins?

   A. Dichorionic diamniotic
   B. Monochorionic diamniotic
   C. Monochorionic monoamniotic
   D. There are no most prevalent structures
   E. None of the above

Answer: B. Monochorionic diamniotic

Comment: Approximately 80% of all **monozygotic twins** are **monochorionic diamniotic**, whereas all **dizygotic twins** are **dichorionic diamniotic**. In other words in all **monochorionic** twin pregnancies twins are **monozygotic**.

Q.25 The incidence of hydatidiform moles is increased in which age group?

   A. 18–20 years
   B. 21–25 years
   C. 26–30 years
   D. 31–40 years
   E. Older than 45 years

Answer: E. Older than 45 years

Comment: **Incidence of hydatidiform moles** (HM) is increased in very young women under the age of **16 years** and those **older than 45 years** of age. The reasons for this age-dependent increased risk are not known. The increased incidence of hydatidiform moles in very young women may account in part for the higher incidence of hydatidiform moles in Asia, Africa, and South America. However, the true reasons for the geographic variation in the incidence of HM are not known. Women who had one molar pregnancy are at increased risk of having another molar pregnancy. Familial forms of HM indicate that genetic factors may play a role in some cases, which are, however, quite rare.

Q.26 What is the karyotype of most complete hydatidiform moles?

   A. 23, X
   B. 23, Y
   C. 46, XX
   D. 46, XY
   E. 69, XXX

Answer: C. 46, XX

Comment: Most **complete hydatidiform moles** (HM) have a 46,XX karyotype. Both sets of chromosomes develop from endoreduplication of a haploid (23,X) sperm, which has entered an ovum devoid of its own (i.e. maternal) chromosomes. This process leading to formation of a **monoparental** conceptus containing only paternal chromosomes is called **androgenesis**. **Biparental** HMs are rare, but clinically important because they occur in an autosomal recessive hereditary form of recurrent HMs. Mutations of a gene called ***NLRP7*** (NACHT, leucine rich repeat, and PYD containing protein 7) on chromosome 19 have been identified as the cause of these HMs. Some microscopic features are more common in recurrent hereditary HM than in sporadic HM, but in general these two genetic types of HM cannot be distinguished microscopically one from another (*Source:* Sabire NJ, et al. Placenta. 2013; 34:50-6).

Q.27 Which of the following karyotypes is most likely found in partial hydatidiform moles?

A. 23, X
B. 23, Y
C. 46, XX
D. 46, XY
E. 69, XXX

Answer: E. 69, XXX

Comment: **Partial moles** are **biparental** and most of them are **triploid**. Triploidy results from fertilization of an ovum with two sperms, which in technical term means that the conceptus is **diandric**. They can be 69, XXX if both fertilizing sperms are 23,X. They also can be 69, XXY, if one sperm carries an X (23,X) and the other a Y chromosome (23, Y). The third possible chromosomal combination (69, XYY) is very rare most likely because it is usually lethal and no parts of the conceptus survive after implantation. One should remember that triploidy does not automatically mean that one is dealing with a partial mole. Tetraploid moles also occur but they are rare and are encountered in 0.7% of all pregnancies (*Source:* Sundvall L, et al. Hum Reprod. 2013;28: 2010-20).

Q.28 Which one of the following microscopic findings favors the diagnosis of first trimester complete hydatidiform mole rather than non-molar products of conception?

A. Basophilic stroma with immature cord-like blood vessels
B. Presence of prominent hematopoietic cells in the villi
C. Absence of stromal cell apoptosis
D. Absence of karyorrhexis of villous endothelial cells
E. Hydropic villi with rounded contours showing polar proliferation of trophoblast

Answer: A. Basophilic stroma with immature blood vessels

Table 5.2: Microscopic features of normal early products of conception, hydropic abortus, and early (first trimester) complete hydatidiform mole

Feature	Normal early POC	Hydropic abortion	Early complete HM
Contours of chorionic villi	Regular round or elongated	Edematous expanded round oval but smooth	Bulbous with deep invaginations
Trophoblast	Two-layered, regular Anchoring villi may have polar proliferation and layering of cells	Stretched and thin No proliferation or layering of cells	Focal polar proliferation and layering of cells Circumferential proliferation later
Stroma of the chorionic villi	Edematous and reticular after 4 weeks	Edematous, clear	Basophilic, may be variable Cisterns form later
Villous vessels	Well-formed lumens	Well-formed lumens	Immature, strand-like with slit-like lumens
Nucleated hematopoietic cells	Present in many early chorionic villi	Scant to absent	Usually absent
Apoptosis/karyorrhexis	Minimal	Minimal	Prominent in both stromal cells and endothelial cells
$p57^{kip2}$—IHC	Normal	Normal	Negative in villi
Short tandem repeat genotyping	Normal	Normal	Androgenesis, proof of 46, XX of paternal origin

Abbreviations: IHC, immunohistochemistry; POC, products of conception; HM, hydatidiform mole.
Source: Kim KR. Gestational trophoblastic disease, Chapter 34. In: Mutter GL, Prat J (Eds). 3rd edition. Pathology of the female reproductive tract. Churchill Livingstone, Elsevier: Edinbourgh; 2014.

Comment: The differential diagnosis of first trimester **complete hydatidiform mole** (CMH), **normal products of conception**, and **hydropic abortus** may be difficult due to the overlapping microscopic features of normal and pathologic placental specimens. In normal products of conception, the anchoring villi are rounded or elongated and show polar proliferation of trophoblast. The same polar proliferation (rather than the circumferential proliferation seen in later stage CHM) may be seen in early CHM, although the villi vary in size and are usually bulbous ("cauliflower-like"). The villous stroma of the normal villi, and hydropic abortus is pale and edematous, containing blood vessels with obvious lumina. In the normal villi, there are also hematopoietic cells and few if any apoptotic bodies. In early CHM, the stroma is basophilic (resembling the villous stroma of the first four weeks of pregnancy) and only later on it becomes hydropic with cistern formation. The blood vessel in the villi of CHM are cord-like and do not have lumina or these may appear slit-like. There are no hematopoietic cells. Apoptotic stromal and vascular cells are prominent. In the final analysis, immunohistochemical staining with the antibody to $p57^{kip2}$ can be useful. Short tandem repeat genotyping could support the diagnosis. Salient differential diagnostic points comparing normal products of conception, hydropic abortion and CHM are presented in the Table 5.2.

Q.29 Immunohistochemistry for $p57^{kip2}$ gave the following results on a placental specimen obtained by curettage in early pregnancy: positive nuclear staining of decidua and extravillous trophoblast and negative staining of chorionic stroma and blood vessels and chorionic trophoblast. These findings are most consistent with which diagnosis?

A. Preeclampsia
B. Complete hydatidiform mole
C. Partial hydatidiform mole
D. Hereditary recurrent mole
E. Invasive mole

Answer: B. Complete hydatidiform mole

Comment: $p57^{kip2}$, officially known as **CDKN1** (cyclin-dependent kinase inhibitor 1C) is a protein encoded by the maternal imprinted *CDKN1C* gene. The protein is also listed in some papers as p57KIP2 or simply p57 (*Source:* Gupta M, et al. Am J Surg Pathol. 2012; 36: 1747-60). Due to its maternal imprinting this gene is not expressed in chorionic villi of **complete hydatidiform mole** (CHM). These villi form, namely, by androgenesis and do not contain any maternal gene products in villous stromal cells and villous trophoblast. Extravillous trophoblastic cells are less restrictive, and thus even in complete moles these cells stain positively with the antibody to $p57^{kip2}$. As one would expect, maternally derived decidual cells express the *CDKN1* gene and could serve as positive control. Partial mole and the hereditary recurrent moles are biparental and contain the active maternal gene, and therefore stain positively with the antibodies to $p57^{kip2}$. This test is accordingly good only for the diagnosis of complete androgenic moles and is not useful for diagnosing hereditary recurrent moles and partial moles.

Q.30 What is the most likely karyotype of the early hydatidiform mole shown in Figure 5.2?

A. 23, X
B. 23, Y
C. 46, XX
D. 46, XY
E. 69, XXX

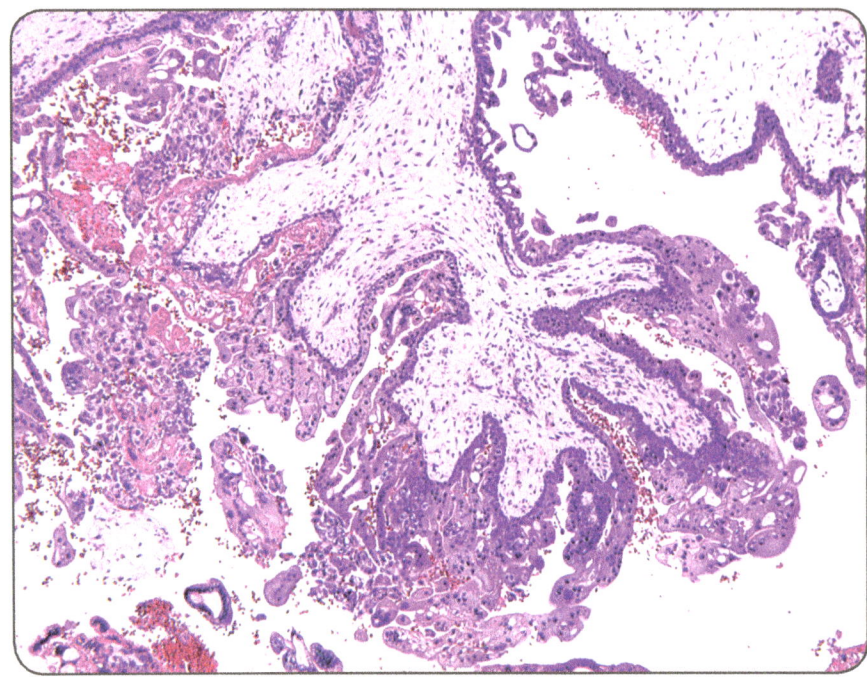

Figure 5.2

Answer: C. 46, XX

Comment: Figure 5.2 shows typical features of complete mole, which has a 46, XX karyotype. These include avascular deeply invaginated villi forming typical "knuckles" covered with proliferating trophoblast.

Q.31 What is the most likely karyotype of this hydatidiform mole shown in Figure 5.3?

- A. 23, X
- B. 23, Y
- C. 46, XX
- D. 46, XY
- E. 69, XXX

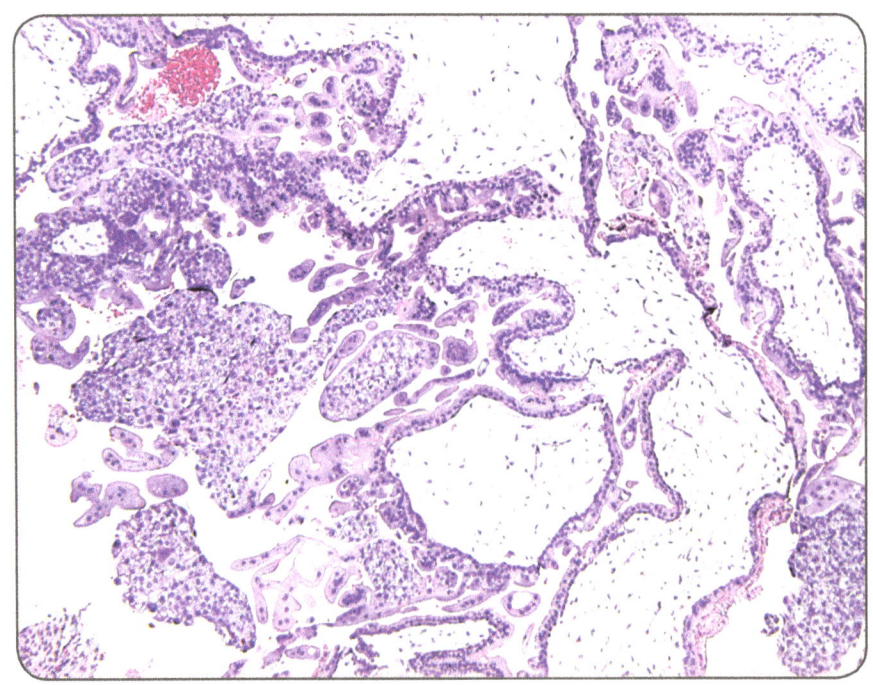

Figure 5.3

Answer: C. 46,XX

Comment: Figure 5.3 shows complete hydatidiform mole. Typical changes include hydropic change of avascular villi containing thin-walled blood vessels with barely visible slit lumens of this 16 weeks old placenta. There is prominent circumferential layering of the proliferated trophoblast on the surface of all villi. Immunohistochemistry for p57^{kip2} was negative on stroma and blood vessels of chorionic villi and chorionic trophoblast, confirming the diagnosis.

Q.32 All the following microscopic findings are typical features of partial hydatidiform moles, *except:*

  A. Extensive circumferential proliferation of villous trophoblast
  B. Angulated and often fibrotic villi admixed with hydropic villi
  C. Central cisterns with angiomatoid stroma
  D. Irregular contours of chorionic villi with deep invaginations
  E. Trophoblastic inclusions in the villi

Answer: A. Extensive circumferential proliferation of villous trophoblast

Comment: The proliferation of villous trophoblast in **partial hydatiform moles** (PHM) is usually mild to moderate and essentially never as prominent as in complete HM. Other features listed here are usually present in PHM. These findings are usually interrelated one to another. For example, the trophoblastic lining of the deep invaginations of the angulated villi may produce an impression of trophoblastic inclusions.

Q.33 Figure 5.4 shows a section from the uterus removed after a complication of pregnancy. What is the most likely diagnosis?

  A. Choriocarcinoma
  B. Complete hydatidiform mole
  C. Partial hydatidiform mole
  D. Hereditary recurrent mole
  E. Invasive mole

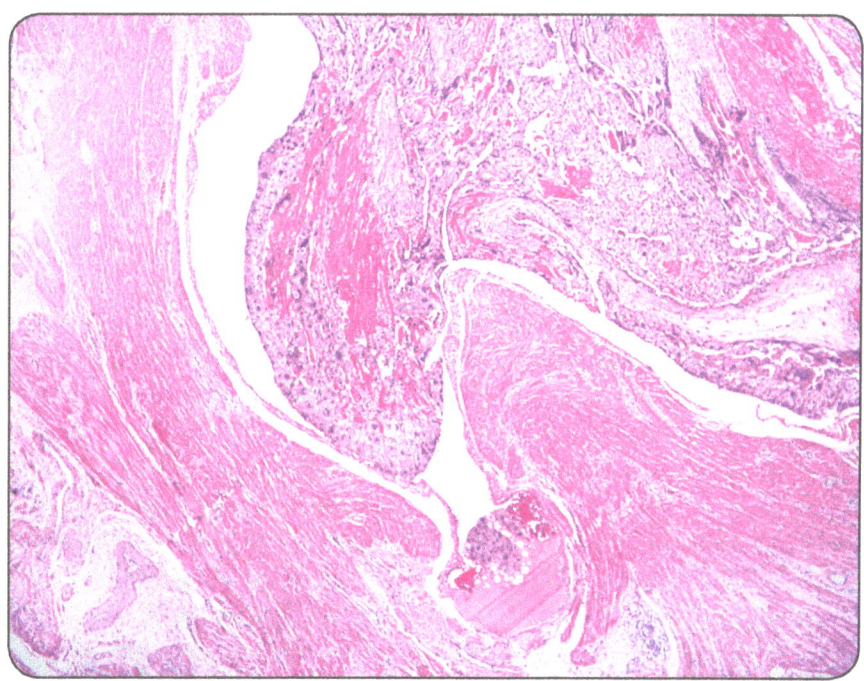

Figure 5.4

Answer: E. Invasive mole

Comment: Figure 5.4 shows invasion of trophoblastic tissue into the myometrium, a typical feature of **invasive mole**.

Q.34 The diagnosis of invasive mole is made most often after which procedure?
   A. Endometrial biopsy
   B. Hysterectomy
   C. Explorative laparotomy
   D. Pulmonary needle biopsy
   E. Liver biopsy

Answer: B. Hysterectomy

Comment: **Invasive mole** is characterized by invasion of trophoblastic tissue into the myometrium or cervical stroma, uterine blood vessels and metastases to distant sites. Most often it is diagnosed in hysterectomy specimens rather than by biopsy, which usually does not contain enough tissue for the final diagnosis. Anatomic documentation of invasive mole is, however, not essential for clinical evaluation and treatment; all patients with persistently high or rising levels of β-hCG in serum detected after the evacuation of a hydatidiform mole will receive chemotherapy for persistent gestational trophoblastic disease.

Q.35 Figure 5.5 shows the microscopic features of an endometrial mass in a hysterectomy specimen following a molar pregnancy. What is the most likely diagnosis?
   A. Choriocarcinoma
   B. Complete hydatidiform mole
   C. Partial hydatidiform mole
   D. Hereditary recurrent mole
   E. Invasive mole

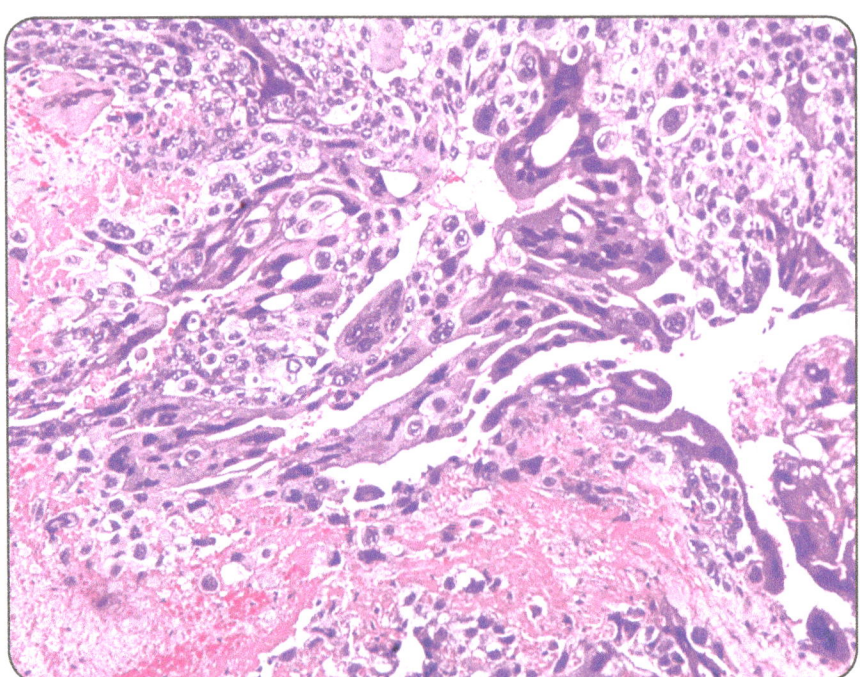

Figure 5.5

Answer: A. Choriocarcinoma

Comment: Figure 5.4 shows the typical features of a choriocarcinoma, which is composed of multinucleated syncytiotrophoblastic cells and mononuclear cytotrophoblastic cells.

Q.36 A 41-year-old woman with clinically diagnosed gestational trophoblastic disease began therapy 14 month after the end of pregnancy. The therapy failed and she was assigned FIGO anatomical staging/FIGO clinical risk factor score of IV:20. What is the most likely extent of this tumor?
   A. Tumor is limited to the uterus
   B. Tumor extends beyond the uterus but is limited to internal genital organs
   C. Tumor has metastasized to spleen or kidney
   D. Tumor has metastasized to the gastrointestinal tract
   E. Tumor has metastasized to the brain, liver

Answer: E. Tumor has metastasized to the brain, liver

Comment: The **FIGO anatomic staging system** on a scale from I to IV is reported in Roman numerals and the **FIGO clinical risk factor score** (0–4 for several variables) is reported in Arabic numbers. Stage IV means distant metastases to any organ except the lungs, which is considered to be still stage III. The number of metastases has to be taken into account for the clinical risk factor score. The number 20 is for example cumulative score of 5 (variables) × 4 (maximal score on the scale from 0 to 4) including metastases to the brain and/or liver, more than 8 metastases, more than 13 month interval between pregnancy and diagnosis, high serum β-hCG, and failed therapy to 2 or more drugs.

Q.37 What is the most common precursor of choriocarcinoma?
   A. Normal pregnancy
   B. Ectopic pregnancy
   C. Abortus
   D. Complete hydatidiform mole
   E. Partial hydatidiform mole

Answer: D. Complete hydatidiform mole

Comment: Approximately, 50% of all **choriocarcinomas** are preceded by hydatidiform moles. Approximately, 80% of those are complete moles. Normal pregnancy precedes choriocarcinoma in 25%, abortions in 22%, and ectopic pregnancies in less than 3% of all cases.

Q.38 All the following components of normal placentation are seen in choriocarcinoma, *except*:
   A. Mononuclear cytotrophoblastic cells
   B. Multinuclear syncytiotrophoblastic cells
   C. Mononuclear intermediate trophoblastic cells
   D. Chorionic villi
   E. b-hCG positive cells

Answer: D. Chorionic villi

Comment: **Choriocarcinoma** are made up of **cytotrophoblastic** and **syncytiotrophoblastic** and less abundant **intermediate trophoblastic** cells, which are usually intermixed one with another. Chorionic villi similar to those in the placenta, are not formed usually, and are not seen except in intraplacental choriocarcinomas, an early form of this tumor confined to the placenta.

Q.39 Placental site trophoblastic tumor is mostly composed of which cells?

  A. Cytotrophoblastic cells
  B. Syncytiotrophoblastic cells
  C. Intermediate trophoblastic cells
  D. Macrophages (Hoffbauer cells)
  E. Angioblasts

Answer: **C. Intermediate trophoblast cells**

Comment: **Placental site trophoblastic tumor** is composed of **intermediate (extravillous) trophoblastic** cells invading the myometrium. These cells are positive for **human placental lactogen** and CD146, the usual markers for intermediate trophoblast. Scattered among these cells one may find syncytiotrophoblastic cells, which account for the mild elevation of β-hCG in serum of these patients.

Q.40 Expressed in percentages, how many placental site trophoblastic tumors are benign?

  A. 10%
  B. 25%
  C. 50%
  D. 66%
  E. 80%

Answer: **E. 80%**

Comment: Most **placental site trophoblastic tumors** are benign but 20% are malignant. The malignant nature of these tumors cannot be predicted on the basis of their microscopic features. Staging is much more important for formulating the prognosis.

CHAPTER 6

Breast

Q.1 What is the most likely diagnosis for this breast biopsy tissue obtained from a 24-year-old woman (Figure 6.1)?

  A. Sclerosing adenosis
  B. Apocrine adenosis
  C. Lactational changes
  D. Apocrine metaplasia
  E. Usual ductal hyperplasia

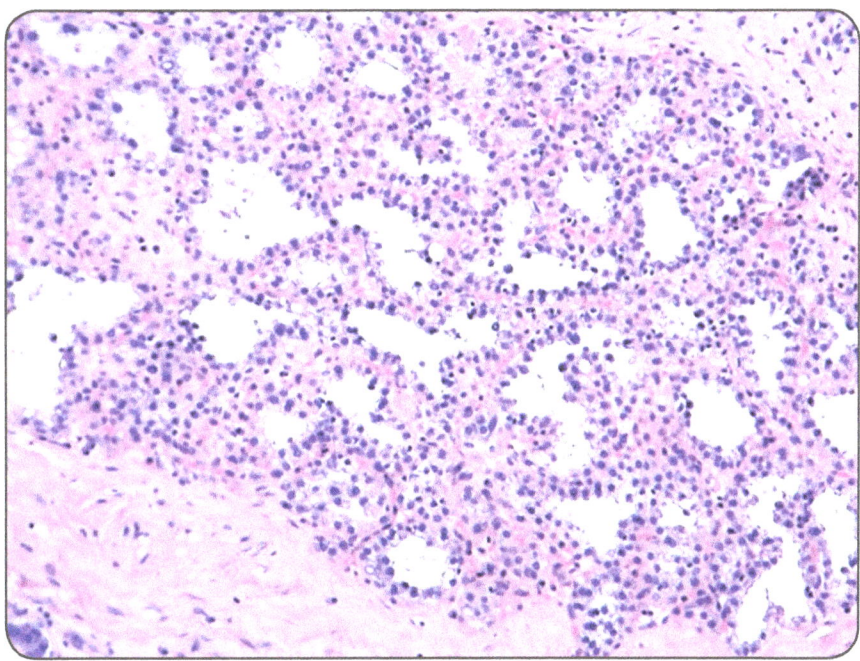

Figure 6.1

Answer: C. Lactational changes

Comment: The Figure shows enlarged lobules and acini which are composed of enlarged epithelial cells showing prominent cytoplasmic vacuolization and a hobnail-like appearance along the luminal border. **Lactational changes** are typically seen during pregnancy and in the postpartum period. If circumscribed, such changes are called lactating adenoma or lactating nodular hyperplasia.

Q.2 Reactive lesions (changes) of the breast related to the prior biopsy site include all, *except*:
   A. Hemorrhage
   B. Duct ectasia
   C. Fat necrosis
   D. Acute or chronic inflammation
   E. Foreign giant body reaction

Answer: B. Duct ectasia

Comment: Changes that are related to a prior biopsy represent the most common reactive lesions in the breast. Apart from the above mentioned changes, the spectrum of reactive changes includes granulation tissue and scarring. **Duct ectasia** is not related to a previous biopsy. It is characterized by a dilatation of large subareolar ducts surrounded by fibrous tissue and chronic inflammatory cells. It is usually found in perimenopausal and postmenopausal women.

Q.3 Breast infarcts occur most often in association with:
   A. Anticoagulant therapy
   B. Intraductal papilloma
   C. Fibroadenoma
   D. Pregnancy
   E. Trauma

Answer: D. Pregnancy

Comment: **Breast infarcts** occur most often during pregnancy or postpartum. They may complicate a large variety of conditions including anticoagulant therapy, inflammatory conditions such as abscesses, sclerosing adenosis and breast tumors such as intraductal papillomas or fibroadenomas. They are not related to breast trauma.

Q.4 Fat necrosis may complicate all of the following conditions, *except*:
   A. Previous surgery
   B. Lactation
   C. Fine needle aspiration biopsy
   D. Trauma
   E. Irradiation therapy

Answer: B. Lactation

Comment: **Fat necrosis** is a well-known mimicker of breast malignancy and is usually associated with previous physical injury of the breast due to trauma, previous surgery, fine-needle aspiration biopsy and irradiation therapy. It is not related to lactation itself, although it may be found in the course of lactation associated infections. It is noteworthy that the cause of fat necrosis in 50% of the cases remains unknown.

Q.5 Apocrine metaplasia of ductal epithelium has all the following immunohistochemical features, *except*:
   A. Estrogen receptor negative (ER-)
   B. Progesterone receptor negative (PR-)
   C. Androgen receptor positive (AR+)
   D. Gross cystic disease fluid protein-15 (GCDFP-15) positive
   E. Basal marker positive (e.g. CK5/6, CK14, p63)

Answer: E. Basal marker positive

Comment: A spectrum of **apocrine lesions** of the breast (from benign to malignant) exhibit a characteristic steroid receptor profile (ER-/PR-/AR+), and are typically positive for GCDFP-15. Although apocrine metaplasia is a benign lesion, it may lack (in part or completely) basal/myoepithelial markers, such as CK5/6, CK14, smooth muscle myosin-heavy chain (SMM-HC), p63, calponin, S-100.

Q.6 **Characteristic morphologic features of mammary duct ectasia include all,** *except:*

- A. Dilated ducts within the terminal duct lobular unit
- B. Periductal inflammation (plasma cells)
- C. Periductal fibrosis
- D. The presence of foamy histiocytes
- E. Obliteration of duct lumens

Answer: **A. Dilated ducts within the terminal duct lobular unit**

Comment: Although, it may be difficult to distinguish duct cysts from duct ectasia, particularly when there is no inflammatory cells, duct ectasia primarily affects extralobular ducts in contrast to cysts that affect the terminal duct lobular units (TDLU). In some cases, special stains highlighting the elastic tissue may be helpful as ducts contain elastic tissue in their walls, which is not the case with the breast cysts.

Q.7 **Which of the following is the most common cause of acute mastitis?**

- A. *Mycobacterium tuberculosis*
- B. *Staphylococcus aureus*
- C. *Staphylococcus epidermidis*
- D. *Histoplasma capsulatum*
- E. *Streptococcus pyogenes*

Answer: **B. *Staphylococcus aureus***

Comment: **Acute (or puerperal) mastitis** usually occurs 2-3 weeks after delivery. It is usually caused by *Staphylococcus aureus,* which is directly transmitted from the skin or the infant. Other streptococci and staphylococci are less common. *Mycobacterium tuberculosis* and *Histoplasma capsulatum* infections occur rarely usually presenting in form of granulomatous mastitis.

Q.8 A 33-year-old woman, two years postpartum, underwent a core needle biopsy of a mass located in upper lateral quadrant of the left breast. The biopsy revealed numerous lobulocentric infiltrates composed of epithelioid macrophages, multinucleated giant cells and lymphocytes. Several special stains for bacteria, mycobacteria and fungi were negative. What is the most likely diagnosis?

- A. Acute mastitis
- B. Sarcoidosis
- C. Foreign giant body reaction
- D. Idiopathic granulomatous mastitis
- E. Duct ectasia

Answer: **D. Idiopathic granulomatous mastitis**

Comment: **Idiopathic granulomatous mastitis** (or lobular granulomatous mastitis) is a rare breast lesion that is typically seen in younger women, usually presenting clinically several month or even years following pregnancy. Microscopically, it is characterized by the lobulocentricity of granulomas. Some lesions also contain neutrophils, often rimming empty spaces formed at the place of washed out lipids. Microabscesses may be seen as well. Caseous necrosis, typical of mycobacterial or fungal infection is not seen.

Q.9 Granulomatous inflammation in the breast may be seen in association with all the following, *except:*

- A. Infections
- B. Foreign material
- C. Systemic diseases
- D. Lymphocytic mastopathy
- E. Carcinomas

Answer: D. Lymphocytic mastopathy

Comment: **Lymphocytic (diabetic) mastopathy** present typically with perivascular and periductal lymphocytic infiltrates, not granulomas. Infections associated with granulomatous reaction include mycobacteria, fungi and parasites while systemic diseases like sarcoidosis may result in epithelioid, non-necrotizing granulomas ("sarcoid-like") similar to those arising elsewhere in the body. Sarcoid-like granulomas may be occasionally seen in the stroma of breast cancers.

Q.10 Key histologic findings in lymphocytic (diabetic) mastopathy include all the following, *except:*

- A. Keloid-like fibrosis
- B. Perivascular lymphocytic infiltrates
- C. Periductal lymphocytic infiltrates
- D. Stromal proliferation
- E. Intraductal epithelial proliferation

Answer: E. Intraductal epithelial proliferation

Comment: **Lymphocytic (diabetic) mastopathy** usually affects young to middle-aged women with previous history of type 1 diabetes mellitus. It usually presents as a symptomatic mass, or several nodule and is often bilateral. It includes all the above mentioned alterations apart from epithelial proliferation. Notably, similar morphologic alterations in the breast may be seen in association with other autoimmune diseases, such as Hashimoto thyroiditis.

Q.11 Squamous metaplasia of the breast may be associated with:

- A. Fibroepithelial tumors
- B. Gynecomastia
- C. Previous trauma
- D. Intraductal papilloma
- E. All of the above

Answer: E. All of the above

Comment: **Squamous metaplasia** of the breast is a rare, reactive change that may be associated with all the above mentioned conditions. In addition, squamous metaplasia may arise within various benign lesions such as cysts and florid ductal hyperplasia.

Q.12 Synovial metaplasia in the breast develops typically in the vicinity of which other finding?

- A. Capsule around silicone containing implants
- B. Ductal carcinoma in situ
- C. Fat necrosis
- D. Duct ectasia
- E. Keloid like scars

Answer: A. Capsule around silicone containing implants

Comment: **Synovial metaplasia**, named so because it resembles the synovial membrane in the joints, is a reactive condition characterized by layering of fibrohistocytic cells positioned perpendicularly to the surface of the membrane. These cells are CD68 and vimentin positive and negative for cytokeratins. The pathogenesis of synovial metaplasia remains unclear. It is assumed that it forms as a reaction to mechanical forces between the implants and adjacent tissue.

Q.13 Complex fibroadenomas of the breast are characterized by all of the following features, *except:*
 A. Increased stromal cellularity
 B. Cysts (larger than 3 mm)
 C. Papillary apocrine metaplasia
 D. Epithelial calcifications
 E. Sclerosing adenosis

Answer: **A. Increased stromal cellularity**

Comment: **Complex fibroadenomas** contain also areas corresponding to sclerosing adenosis, papillary apocrine hyperplasia, cysts or epithelial calcification. Increased stromal cellularity (also known as stromal hypercellularity) is not a feature of complex fibroadenomas; it is a diagnostic feature of phyllodes tumors of the breast but may also be seen in juvenile (giant) fibroadenomas that typically affect adolescents and young girls. Phyllodes tumors also exhibit other gross and microscopic characteristics that may help distinguish two types of fibroepithelial tumors of the breast. Women with complex fibroadenomas are at a higher risk for breast cancer than those who have classical fibroadenomas.

Q.14 A mobile well-circumscribed palpable mass measuring approximately 3 cm in diameter was identified in a 26-year-old woman. The lesion was biopsied (Figure 6.2). What is the most likely diagnosis?
 A. Phyllodes tumor
 B. Complex fibroadenoma
 C. Juvenile/cellular fibroadenoma
 D. Fibroadenoma
 E. Periductal stromal tumor

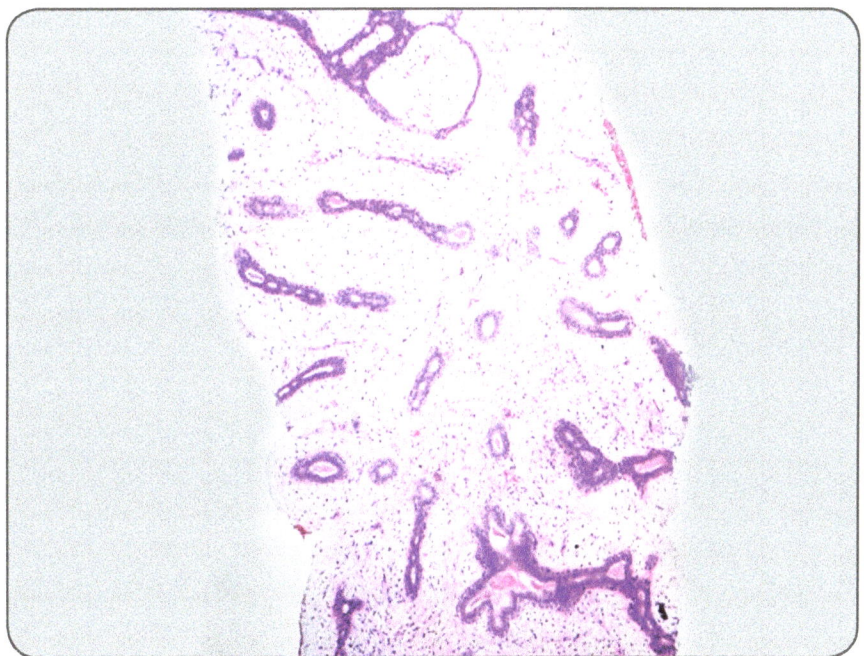

Figure 6.2

Answer: D. Fibroadenoma

Comment: Figure 6.2 shows a mammary **fibroadenoma**, a benign tumor composed of glandular and stromal elements. The stroma may vary from one lesion to another, but it is typically uniform within each particular tumor.
Phyllodes tumor can be excluded because the stroma is not hypercellular and the stroma to epithelium ratio is not increased. Furthermore, the stromal cells do not form fascicles and do not show nuclear atypia or mitotic activity. Most phyllodes tumors show considerable stromal heterogeneity.
Complex fibroadenomas usually affect older patients and contain cysts (>3 mm in size), sclerosing adenosis, calcifications and/or apocrine changes.
Juvenile (cellular) fibroadenomas usually present in adolescents under the age of 20 years and show prominent stromal hypercellularity that is not seen here.
Periductal stromal tumors are characterized by atypical spindle cell proliferation around open ducts.

Q.15 Myxoid changes within a mammary fibroadenoma ("myxoid fibroadenoma") are commonly seen in the patients with:

   A. Cowden syndrome
   B. Carney syndrome
   C. Fanconi anemia
   D. Ataxia-telangiectasia
   E. Peutz-Jeghers syndrome

Answer: B. Carney syndrome

Comment: **Myxoid fibroadenomas** are typically seen in patients with **Carney syndrome**. Cowden syndrome is associated with *PTEN* gene mutations and these patients may develop breast cancers with apocrine differentiation. Patients with Fanconi anemia, ataxia-telangiectasia and Peutz-Jeghers syndromes are at increased risk for breast cancer (approximately 2–4 × increased risk), but do not develop myxoid fibroadenomas.

Q.16 Expressed in percentages, how many fibroadenomas undergo malignant transformation?

   A. 0.1%
   B. 1%
   C. 2%
   D. 5%
   E. 10%

Answer: A. 0.1%

Comment: **Malignant transformation of fibroadenomas** is very rare, occurring in only ~0.1% of all tumors. These rare malignancies are usually of epithelial rather than stromal origin.

Q.17 What is the appropriate surgical margin for phyllodes tumors?

   A. 1 mm
   B. 2 mm
   C. 5 mm
   D. 10 mm
   E. None of the above

Answer: E. None of the above

Comment: Clean **surgical margins** are clinically relevant for the management and prognosis of the patients with **borderline and malignant phyllodes tumors**. However, there is no consensus at the moment for the appropriate margin width. A recent consensus review suggested a pragmatic approach that considers the tumor cells on ink or <1 mm as a positive margin (*Source:* Tan BY, et al. Histopathology. 2016; 68:5-21). Several previous studies considered margins to be positive if the tumor cells are <10 mm from the ink.

Q.18 Mammary hamartoma (Figure 6.3) is composed of various tissues including all the following, *except:*

- A. Fibrous stroma
- B. Adipose tissue
- C. Adenosis
- D. Ducts
- E. Lobules

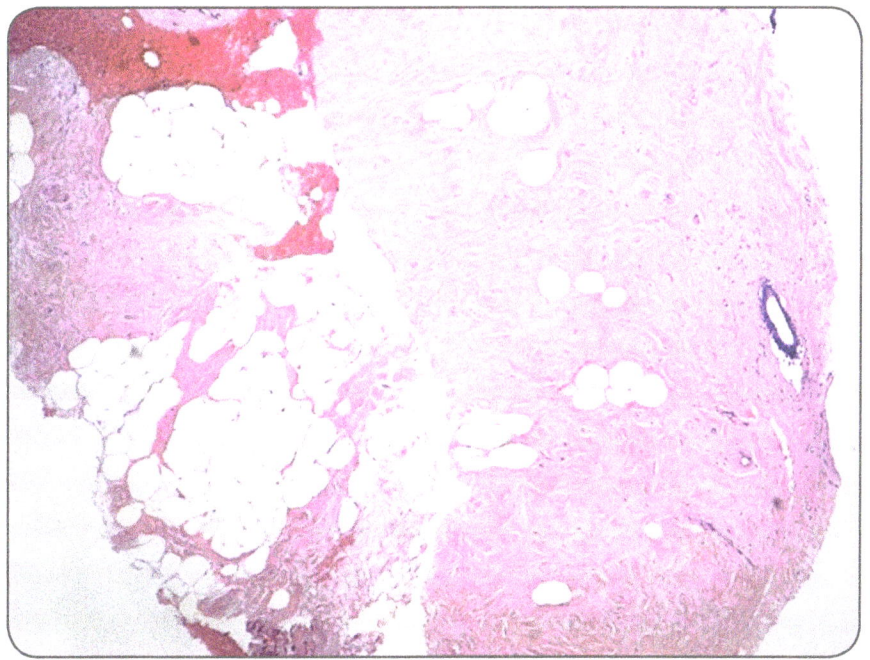

Figure 6.3

Answer: C. Adenosis

Comment: **Mammary hamartomas** are entirely benign, unencapsulated breast lesions that may mimic fibroepithelial tumors (both clinically and radiologically). All the components within the hamartoma are haphazardly distributed resembling normal breast tissue and therefore it can be hardly diagnosed without clinical and radiologic findings. However, any type of adenosis, such as sclerosing adenosis within complex fibroadenomas, or fibrocystic change, is not seen in hamartomas.

Q.19 What is the most likely diagnosis for the tumor shown in Figure 6.4?

- A. Tubular adenoma
- B. Pleomorphic adenoma
- C. Fibroadenoma
- D. Phyllodes tumor
- E. Adenomyoepithelioma

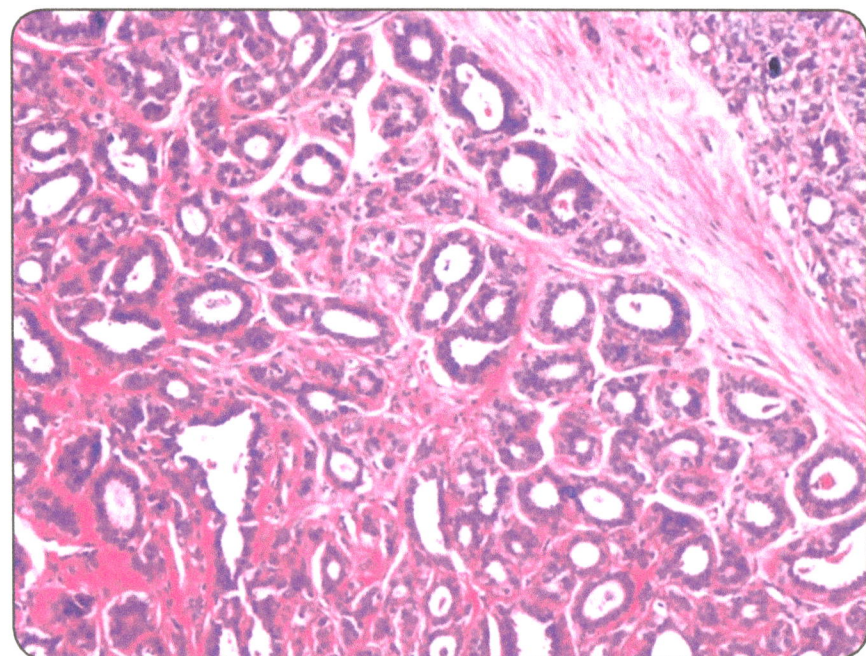

Figure 6.4

Answer: E. Adenomyoepithelioma

Comment: Figure 6.4 shows an **adenomyoepithelioma**, a well-circumscribed tumor, composed of coexistent proliferation of both breast tubules (luminal) and myoepithelial cells, which is a diagnostic clue to adenomyoepithelioma. Proliferation of myoepithelial component may be prominent and this can be confirmed by the myoepithelial/basal markers (e.g. cytokeratins 5/6 and 14; p63, calponin, smooth muscle actin (SMA), H-caldesmon). Tubular adenoma may show similar pattern, but the proliferation of myoepithelial cells is not evident. Pleomorphic adenomas are rare primary tumors in the breast and these typically contain chondroid or myxoid stroma with/without chondroid/osseous metaplasia (similar to their salivary gland counterparts).

Q.20 Which of the following histopathologic features of fibrocystic changes must be properly evaluated to exclude atypical ductal hyperplasia?

    A. Papillary apocrine metaplasia
    B. Intraductal hyperplasia
    C. Sclerosing adenosis
    D. Fibrosis
    E. Cysts

Answer: B. Intraductal hyperplasia

Comment: **Intraductal hyperplasia** (proliferation) is the most critical morphologic feature of fibrocystic change because pathologists must distinguish between usual ductal hyperplasia (UDH) from atypical ductal hyperplasia (ADH). ADH is associated with increased risk of breast cancer. In the challenging cases, immunohistochemical markers (basal cytokeratins, myoepithelial markers as well as the pattern of Estrogen receptor expression) may help rendering the correct diagnosis.

Q.21 Which of the following is a key feature of sclerosing adenosis?

   A. Infiltrative, non-lobulocentric proliferation of small glands
   B. Lobulocentric glands entrapped by fibrous or fibroelastotic connective tissue
   C. Common involvement by in situ and invasive carcinoma
   D. A palpable mass
   E. The lack of calcifications

Answer: B. Lobulocentric glands entrapped by fibrous or fibroelastotic connective tissue

Comment: Sclerosing adenosis is a lobulocentric proliferation of small entrapped glands and tubules and is typically an incidental finding. In contrast, a rare variant of adenosis named microglandular adenosis (MGA) represents a nonlobulocentric, infiltrative lesion with non-compressed glands. MGA also presents as a palpable mass. Both lesions may have calcifications, but morphologically and immunohistochemically MGA lacks myoepithelial cell layer. Sclerosing adenosis is rarely affected by in situ and invasive carcinoma (both ductal and lobular) while MGA, particularly atypical variants, may be associated with a subset of aggressive triple-negative breast carcinomas with basal features as their non-obligate precursor.

Q.22 Apocrine adenosis is a variant of:

   A. Microglandular adenosis
   B. Tubular adenosis
   C. Sclerosing adenosis
   D. Blunt duct adenosis
   E. Secretory adenosis

Answer: C. Sclerosing adenosis

Comment: **Apocrine adenosis** is a variant of sclerosing adenosis in which the cells exhibit a characteristic apocrine morphology: Abundant, eosinophilic, granular cytoplasm and large nuclei with prominent nucleoli. Its variant atypical apocrine adenosis denotes a lesion with the prominent apocrine atypia (at least a three-fold increase in nuclear size and nuclear enlargement). This lesion may be diagnostically challenging with apocrine DCIS involving sclerosing adenosis.

Q.23 Radial scar lesion and complex sclerosing lesions of the breast show a significant morphologic overlap that includes all features, *except*:

   A. Stromal fibrosis and fibroelastosis with entrapped ducts/glands
   B. Preserved basal/myoepithelial cell layer
   C. Varying degree of proliferation and cystic changes in peripheral ducts/lobules
   D. Radial scar lesions are usually larger than complex sclerosing lesions
   E. Complex sclerosing lesions do not show a well-defined radial growth pattern

Answer: D. Radial scar lesions are usually larger than complex sclerosing lesions

Comment: **Radial scar** and complex sclerosing lesion belong to the category of sclerosing lesions of the breast with a significant morphologic overlap and similarity. The most authors agree that complex sclerosing lesions tend to be larger compared with radial scar lesion and exhibit a less-defined radial growth pattern. Some authors believe that complex sclerosing lesions represent a late stage of intraductal papilloma with extensive sclerosis. Both lesions may mimic breast cancer mammographically and clinically. These lesions can be cured by a conservative surgery in the absence of coexistent atypical proliferation (e.g. in situ or invasive carcinoma).

Q.24 Which of the following entities *is not* a variant of intraductal papilloma?

   A. Collagenous spherulosis
   B. Ductal adenoma
   C. Adenomyoepithelioma
   D. Pleomorphic adenoma
   E. None of the above

Answer: **A. Collagenous spherulosis**

Comment: Although, **collagenous spherulosis** may be seen within an intraductal papilloma, it is a distinct entity that may also be seen in a variety of proliferative breast lesions including florid ductal hyperplasia, atypical ductal hyperplasia, radial scar lesion, adenosis, etc. It is usually an incidental finding quite distinct from breast malignancies such as DCIS, adenoid cystic carcinoma or signet ring carcinoma. Other entities listed here (ductal adenoma, pleomorphic adenoma, adenomyoepithelioma) are rare, benign tumors, usually considered to be variants of **intraductal papillomas**.

Q.25 Figure 6.5 of the core biopsy of the nipple lesion in a 58-year-old woman with clinical diagnosis of Paget disease shows the following characteristics, *except*:

   A. Glandular proliferation
   B. Prominent papillary hyperplasia
   C. Involvement of overlying epidermis
   D. Usual ductal hyperplasia
   E. Increased pleomorphism and mitotic activity

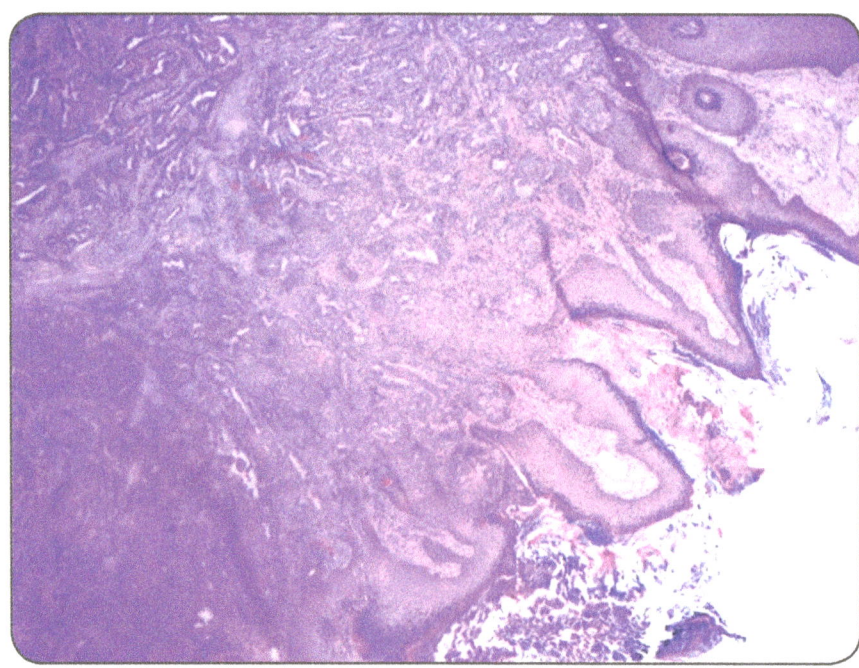

Figure 6.5

Answer: E. Increased pleomorphism and mitotic activity

Comment: The lesion corresponds to a **nipple adenoma** (florid papillomatosis of the nipple). Although, it may clinically mimic **Paget disease**, it is a completely benign lesion. Rare cases of recurrence have been reported due to the incomplete resection. Cell atypia and mitotic activity that are features of Paget disease are rarely encountered in the nipple adenoma. Differential diagnosis also includes **syringomatous adenoma**, which presents usually as an infiltrative lesion, composed of small glands, solid nests and squamous cysts.

Q.26 All the statements regarding tubular adenoma are correct, *except:*
- A. Affects young adults
- B. Solitary lesion
- C. Well-circumscribed
- D. Variant of nipple adenoma
- E. Variant of fibroadenoma

Answer: D. Variant of nipple adenoma

Comment: **Tubular adenoma** is a rare variant of **fibroadenoma**, and not a nipple adenoma. It is composed of tightly packed small tubules. Similar to fibroadenoma, it usually affects young females and has a radiologic and gross features of fibroadenoma.

Q.27 Which of the following entities is not a biphasic fibroepithelial lesion?
- A. Syringomatous tumor
- B. Fibroadenoma
- C. Adenolipoma
- D. Hamartoma
- E. Phyllodes tumor

Answer: A. Syringomatous tumor

Comments: Fibroepithelial tumors of the breast are a heterogeneous group of biphasic tumors (stromal and epithelial) that primarily includes fibroadenomas and phyllodes tumors (benign and malignant). Hamartoma (or adenolipoma) are not strictly fibroepithelial tumors but are usually included in the fibroepithelial group due do the clinical, radiological and histological similarities with fibroadenomas. Syringomatous tumor is a locally aggressive epithelial neoplasm of nipple/areola complex showing sweat-duct differentiation.

Q.28 A 2 cm well-circumscribed tumor was removed from the lateral upper quadrant of breast of a 60 year-old woman. The neoplastic spindle cells (Figure 6.6) were positive for CD34 and smooth muscle cell actin. No mitoses were identified and there was no necrosis. What is the best diagnosis?
- A. Leiomyoma
- B. Fibromatosis
- C. Spindle cell metaplastic carcinoma
- D. Myofibrosarcoma
- E. Myofibroblastoma

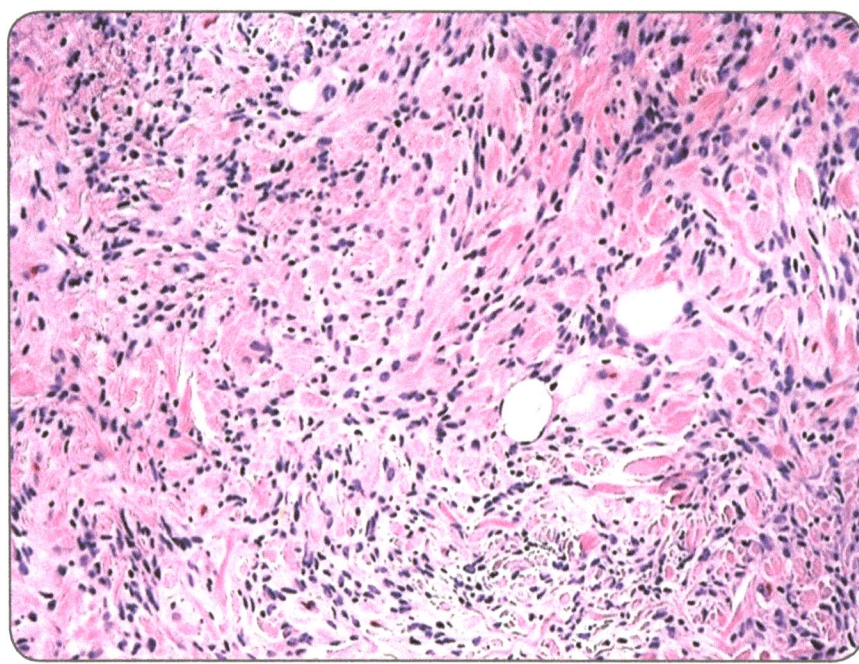

Figure 6.6

Answer: E. Myofibroblastoma

Comment: The photomicrograph shows a neoplasm composed of spindle cells forming fascicles rimmed thick bands of dense collagen. These morphologic features are seen in mammary **myofibroblastoma**. In contrast, fibromatosis is a locally infiltrative lesion composed of long fascicles of bland spindle cells. Spindle cell carcinoma and myofibrosarcoma exhibit morphologic features of malignancy including cellular atypia, pleomorphism, increased mitotic activity and tumor necrosis. Spindle cell lesions of the breast require a thorough work-up with a comprehensive immunohistochemical examination to rule out malignancies, such as metaplastic carcinoma or malignant phyllodes tumor.

Q.29 All the following are typical features of florid (usual) ductal hyperplasia, *except*:

- A. Ductal proliferation creating irregular lumens
- B. Minimal variation in cell size and shape
- C. Bridges are stretched or twisted
- D. Mixed cell population
- E. Cell borders poorly defined

Answer: B. Minimal variation in cell size and shape

Comment: **Usual ductal hyperplasia** (UDH) is considered to be a benign epithelial proliferation distinct from atypical ductal hyperplasia (ADH). ADH has in part a monoclonal cell population that shares some features of low-grade ductal carcinoma in situ (DCIS). ADH cells are typically small, uniform cells with round nuclei (minimal variation in cell size and shape); the cell population is evenly spaced and has well-defined borders. The distinction ADH vs. DCIS is somehow subjective and arbitrary and is based on the size of the lesion and its extent (e.g. 2 mm cut-off and/or 2 ducts involved by atypical intraductal proliferation).

Q.30 All the following are common microscopic subtypes of ductal carcinoma in situ (DCIS), *except*:

- A. Comedo
- B. Cribriform
- C. Solid

D. Cystic
E. Papillary
F. Micropapillary

Answer: **D. Cystic**

Comment: All the above mentioned patterns of **DCIS** are frequently seen except for the cystic variant, which is rare and usually a part of the **cystic hypersecretory DCIS.** Hypersecretory DCIS is composed of multiple cysts filled with homogenous, thyroid-like eosinophilic material.

Other rare types of DCIS include those with apocrine, squamous, clear cell, signet ring, mucinous, endocrine, and spindle cell features.

Of note, a three-tiered system based primarily on nuclear grade and/or necrosis has been developed and validated for clinical practice. This system stratifies DCIS into three grades: low, intermediate, and high-grade DCIS. Further advancements in molecular pathology of DCIS will move its classification toward a specific (molecular) approach.

Q.31 Which of the following biomarkers is routinely evaluated in the patients with DCIS?

A. p53 protein
B. Ki-67 (MIB-1)
C. Estrogen receptor (ER)
D. Progesterone receptor (PR)
E. Her2/neu

Answer: **C. Estrogen receptor**

Comment: Only **estrogen receptor** (ER) has been approved for routine evaluation although many diagnostic laboratories routinely provide a complete immunohistochemical panel analog to the one for invasive breast cancer (ER, PR, Her2/neu, Ki-67/MIB-1). Some pathologists also routinely do basal markers (CK5/6, EGFR) to provide the molecular classification of DCIS [Luminal (A and B), basal-like, triple-negative].

Q.32 What is the risk for invasive mammary carcinoma in a patient who had a biopsy diagnosis of atypical ductal hyperplasia?

A. Not more than fibrocystic disease
B. 3–5x
C. 6–7x
D. 8–10x
E. 11–14

Answer: **B. 3–5x**

Comment: **ADH bears a risk** of subsequent breast cancer (3–5x), which is significantly lower than the risk for low-grade DCIS (8–10x). **DCIS** typically recurs at the same site (either as DCIS or invasive breast cancer) and the treatment options are strikingly different (surgery plus tamoxifen for DCIS vs. follow-up with/without tamoxifen). Axillary lymph node dissection is not relevant for management for either lesion although a subset of DCIS patients may have lymph node metastases that have been shown to be clinically irrelevant.

Q.33 Features that are associated with increased risk of recurrence of ductal carcinoma in situ (DCIS) following breast-conserving surgery include all, *except:*

A. Patient's age (<45 years)
B. Comedo-necrosis
C. Surgical margins
D. Nuclear atypia
E. Histotype of DCIS

Answer: E. Histotype of DCIS

Comment: Patients diagnosed with **ductal carcinoma in situ (DCIS)** and treated with breast-conserving surgery are at increased risk of local recurrence (50% of recurrences are in a form of invasive carcinoma. The most important factor associated with recurrence of DCIS is a status of surgical margins. The optimal distance of tumor cells to the surgical margins is still under debate and remains to be defined. Several predictive models (e.g. the University of Southern California-Van Nuys Prognostic Index, USC-VNPI) have been developed to stratify the patients with DCIS in regards to the risk of recurrence, but they still require a full clinical validation. Histotype of DCIS may be associated with some of the above mentioned parameters used for the assessment of DCIS, but is not crucial for patient's prognosis.

Q.34 The term extensive intraductal carcinoma in situ implies the presence of DCIS in more than:

A. 25% of tumor volume
B. 50% of tumor volume
C. 10% of tumor volume
D. 75% of tumor volume
E. 90% of tumor volume

Answer: A. 25% of tumor volume

Comment: Extensive **DCIS** is proposed for breast cancers in which in situ component comprises ≥25% of the tumor. Extensive DCIS is usually a high-grade cancer.

Q.35 What is the best diagnosis for the lesion shown in Figure 6.7?

A. Cystic hypersecretory DCIS
B. Apocrine DCIS
C. Invasive apocrine carcinoma
D. Apocrine metaplasia

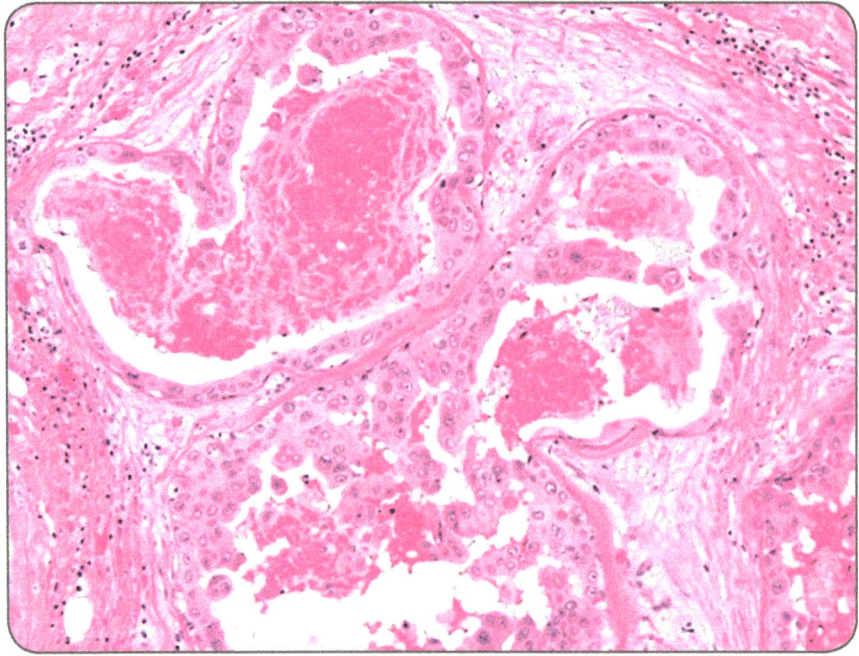

Figure 6.7

Answer: B. Apocrine DCIS

Comment: The Figure shows two adjacent ducts lined by highly atypical epithelial cells with apocrine morphology; both ducts have a central comedo necrosis. These findings are consistent with **apocrine DCIS**. Adjacent tissue contained invasive component with similar morphology (not shown). Apocrine metaplasia is a common, benign finding, frequently seen in patients with fibrocystic changes. Cystic hypersecretory DCIS is a rare form of DCIS, with cysts lined by flattened, not apocrine epithelium and intraluminal secretions.

Q.36 Histologic criteria that may help for distinguishing lobular carcinoma in situ (LCIS) from low-grade, solid variant of ductal carcinoma in situ (DCIS) include all the following, *except:*

- A. Loss of cohesion
- B. Pagetoid spread
- C. Intracytoplasmic vacuoles ("signet ring" appearance)
- D. Mitotic activity
- E. Microacini

Answer: D. Mitotic activity

Comment: None of the above mentioned features is specific enough but mitotic activity is generally low in both **low-grade solid DCIS and LCIS** and consequently not reliable feature to distinguish between DCIS and LCIS. In equivocal cases, immunohistochemical markers such as E-cadherin, β-catenin, p120 catenin, and high-molecular weight cyto-keratins (e.g. 34βE12) may be particularly helpful. Both LCIS and DCIS typically overexpress estrogen receptor (ER-α).

Q.37 A small subset of invasive breast carcinomas associated with atypical microglandular adenosis shows the following features:

- A. Alveolar growth pattern
- B. Clear cytoplasm of the tumor cells
- C. Preponderance of special histologic types
- D. Triple-negative phenotype
- E. Positivity for S-100 protein

Answer: C. Preponderance of special histologic types

Comment: **Microglandular adenosis** is a rare breast lesion that has been recently recognized as a non-obligate precursor of invasive breast carcinoma. The vast majority of these carcinomas are no-special-type (NST). Rare cases of special histologic types (e.g. adenoid cystic carcinoma, metaplastic carcinoma) associated with microglandular adenosis have also been described. Notably, invasive carcinomas associated with microglandular adenosis typically exhibit a triple-negative phenotype (ER/PR/Her2) and S-100 positivity analogue to the immunohistochemical profile of microglandular adenosis.

Q.38 Intraductal papilloma and papillomatosis may be distinguished from papillary DCIS on the basis of all the features below, *except:*

- A. Cell types and orientation
- B. Size
- C. Nuclei appearance
- D. Stroma
- E. Apocrine metaplasia

Answer: B. Size

Comment: **Intraductal papillomas** typically have a dual cell population composed of normochromatic epithelial (luminal) and myoepithelial (basal cells) within a prominent stroma in contrast to papillary DCIS. Apocrine metaplasia frequently accompanies benign papillary lesions including intraductal papilloma. The size of the lesion is not a reliable distinguishing characteristic. It may be relevant for the discrimination between intraductal papilloma with atypia (i.e. atypical papilloma) and DCIS arising in a papilloma (≥3 mm atypical focus is a cut-off according to the 2011, WHO Working Group), which must be distinguished from papillary DCIS.

Q.39 Lobular carcinoma in situ (LCIS) is characterized by the following clinical characteristics, *except:*

- A. Primarily found in postmenopausal women
- B. Commonly an incidental finding
- C. Prone to multicentricity and multifocality
- D. Bilateral in approximately 30% of the cases
- E. Associated with 8-10 fold invasive breast carcinoma risk

Answer: **A. Primarily found in postmenopausal women**

Comment: LCIS typically (80-90%) affects premenopausal, rather than postmenopausal women. The mean age of women diagnosed with LCIS is 45 years. LCIS is prone to be multifocal (~70%) and bilateral (~30%).

Q.40 Patients with lobular carcinoma in situ (LCIS) are at increased risk of invasive breast carcinoma. What is the estimated risk?

- A. 2-4x
- B. 4-6x
- C. 6-8x
- D. 8-10x
- E. 15-17x

Answer: D. 8-10x

Comment: Approximately, 20-30% patients with diagnosed **lobular carcinoma in situ** (LCIS) will develop invasive breast cancer, which implies 8-10x increased risk of breast cancer in comparison with the general population.

Q.41 Columnar cell lesions of the breast show all of the following characteristics, *except:*

- A. Apical snouts
- B. Increased mitotic activity
- C. Columnar cell appearance
- D. Intraluminal secretions
- E. Calcifications (psammoma bodies)

Answer: B. Increased mitotic activity

Comment: **Columnar cell lesions** have been increasingly detected due to the calcifications detected by mammography. Previously, their classification was complex and inconsistent, but now a more consistent and applicable classification has been adopted. It includes columnar cell changes, columnar cell hyperplasia and flat epithelial atypia (FEA). Although, these lesions may occasionally show mitotic figures, they typically have a low mitotic activity including low MIB-1 index (Ki-67 staining).

Q.42 What is the best diagnosis for the breast lesion shown in Figure 6.8?
  A. Florid intraductal hyperplasia
  B. DCIS
  C. Flat epithelial atypia (FEA)
  D. Atypical lobular hyperplasia
  E. Sclerosing adenosis

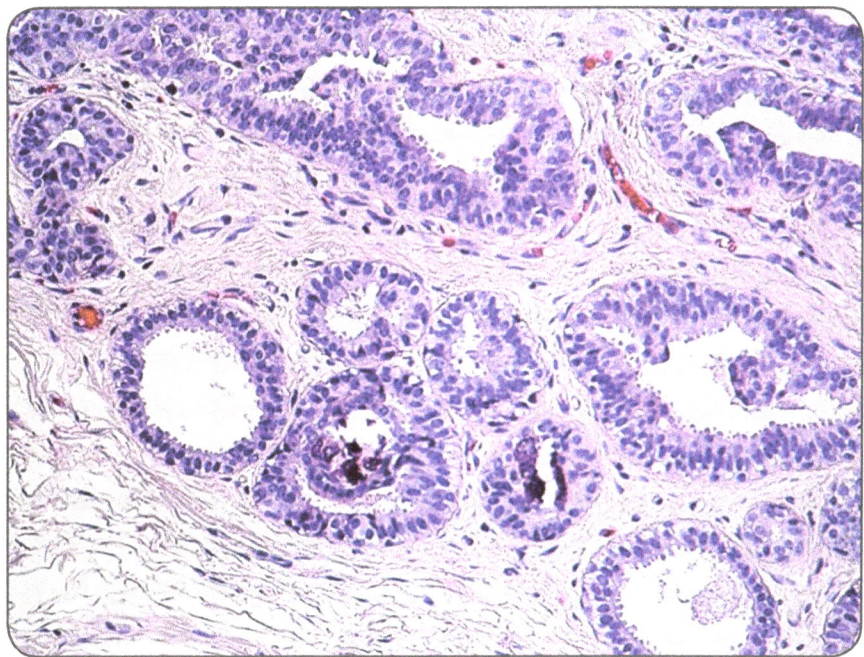

Figure 6.8

Answer: **C. Flat epithelial atypia**

Comment: The Figure shows foci of columnar cell changes and hyperplasia with mild to moderate cellular atypia, diagnostic of **flat epithelial atypia** (FEA). Note the presence of calcifications within the foci of columnar proliferation. Although, FEA may be associated with lobular neoplasia including ALH it is not present in Figure 6.8. FEA morphology may be similar to that of low-grade ductal carcinoma in situ, but usually lacks complex proliferative changes such as bridges, arcades and micropapillae.

Q.43 The "Rosen's triad" includes the following breast lesions, *except:*
  A. Lobular carcinoma in situ (LCIS)
  B. Columnar cell lesions [Flat epithelial atypia (FEA)]
  C. Tubular carcinoma
  D. Invasive lobular carcinoma

Answer: **D. Invasive lobular carcinoma**

Comment: Several studies confirmed an association between **flat epithelial atypia (FEA), lobular carcinoma in situ (LCIS), and tubular carcinoma,** so called "Rosen's triad". The morphologic observations were also confirmed by molecular genetic studies. Some recent studies clustered invasive lobular and **low-grade ductal carcinoma in situ (DCIS)** in the same genetic pathway of "low-grade breast cancer".

Q.44 Approximately, 50% of breast carcinomas are located in which part of the breast?

    A. Lower outer quadrant
    B. Upper outer quadrant
    C. Lower inner quadrant
    D. Upper inner quadrant
    E. Retroareolar region

Answer: **B. Upper outer quadrant**

Comment: **Upper outer quadrant** is the most common location of primary breast carcinoma (~50%) while all other quadrants including central portion (retroareolar region) are affected in approximately 50%.

Q.45 Mammography cannot detect breast tumors that smaller than:

    A. 5 mm
    B. 10 mm
    C. 1–2 mm
    D. 8 mm
    E. 1 cm

Answer: **C. 1–2 mm**

Comment: Mammography can detect very **small tumors** (1-2 mm), particularly those affecting postmenopausal women. Mammography is of particular relevance if microcalcifications are visible (present).

Q.46 Calcium oxalate crystals detected on mammogram are suggestive of:

    A. Intraductal carcinoma
    B. Invasive carcinoma
    C. Benign cysts with apocrine epithelium
    D. Intraductal papilloma
    E. Fibroadenoma

Answer: **C. Benign cysts with apocrine epithelium**

Comment: **Calcium oxalate crystals** have low to medium density and are typically seen in benign breast with cysts lined by apocrine type of epithelium. Calcium phosphate deposits usually have high to medium density, irregular shapes, and are more frequently associated with breast cancer (both in in-situ and invasive). Intraductal papilloma may also have calcifications but has a distinct clinical and radiologic presentation while fibroadenomas are rarely presented with calcifications.

Q.47 Needle core biopsy (NCB) is not conclusive in diagnosis of the following condition:

    A. Atypical ductal hyperplasia
    B. Atypical lobular hyperplasia
    C. Radial scar lesion
    D. Intraductal papilloma
    E. All of the above

Answer: **E. All of the above**

Comment: Needle core biopsy (NCB) is a standard for breast cancer diagnostics with an excellent concordance with surgical biopsies. However, NCB has several limitations and these include the above mentioned entities (diagnosis) as well as some other, rare lesions (e.g. mucocele-like lesion, fibroepithelial tumors with stromal proliferation, spindle cell lesions, etc.). When a definitive diagnosis is not possible on NBC, the appropriate classification includes descriptive terms such as "borderline", "suspicious" or "uncertain malignant potential" (B categories 3-4).

Q.48 Pathology category classification B3 includes all the conditions listed below, *except*:
   A. Papillary lesions
   B. Atypical lobular hyperplasia
   C. Fat necrosis
   D. Phyllodes tumors
   E. Columnar lesions

Answer: **C. Fat necrosis**

Comment: Pathology category classification is widely used by the UK National Health Service Breast Screening Program (NHSBSP) and some other mammographic screening programs (e.g. Australian). It includes five categories (B1 = normal tissue; B2 = benign tissue; B3 = Lesion of uncertain malignant potential; B4 = Suspicious and B5 = malignant/5a = in situ; 5b = invasive). All the above mentioned entities belong to the B3 category except fat necrosis that is classified as B2 (benign).

Q.49 Multicentricity is most commonly seen in which form of breast carcinoma?
   A. Ductal carcinoma NOS
   B. Papillary carcinoma
   C. Lobular carcinoma
   D. Mucinous carcinoma
   E. Tubular carcinoma

Answer: **C. Lobular carcinoma**

Comment: **Multicentricity in breast cancer** is defined by presence of invasive cancer in one or more quadrants other than the one containing the dominant (largest) mass. Multicentricity is typically seen in patients with **lobular carcinoma** and is less common in ductal of NOS and special types such as papillary and mucinous carcinoma.

Q.50 Breast carcinoma is considered to be synchronous when a contralateral breast carcinoma is detected within:
   A. 1 month
   B. 3 months
   C. 6 months
   D. 12 months
   E. 5 years

Answer: **B. 3 months**

Comment: 3 months is usually considered as a period for **synchronous tumors** while tumors are considered metachronous if contralateral breast cancer is diagnosed after more 3 months upon detection (diagnosis) of the first tumor. Certainly, the diagnosis of synchronous breast tumors may be only rendered if metastatic cancer to the contralateral breast is excluded.

Q.51 What is the most important single prognostic factor in breast cancers?

- A. Tumor size
- B. Tumor grade
- C. Molecular subtype
- D. Status of axillary lymph nodes
- E. Histotype

Answer: **D. Status of axillary lymph nodes**

Comment: Although, all the above mentioned parameters are relevant for the treatment and prognosis, the **status of axillary lymph nodes** has been confirmed to be the most relevant prognosticator. It strongly correlates with the tumor size but not necessarily with other parameters (histo- and molecular subtypes and tumor grade).

Q.52 What percentage of tubules within the invasive breast cancer implies a score 1 according to the modified Nottingham histologic grading?

- A. >50%
- B. >75%
- C. > 70%
- D. > 10%
- E. 10–70%

Answer: B. >75%

Comment: **The Nottingham histologic grading** (Elson and Ellis modification of Bloom and Richardson grading system) is recommended for routine evaluation of all invasive breast cancers including special types. It includes the evaluation of the tubules, nuclear grade, and mitotic figures (1–3 point for each). The tumor with > 75% tubule formations gets a score 1 for tubules, 10–75% score 2, and <10% score 3.

Q.53 Which tissue compartment should be most meticulously evaluated for lymphovascular invasion?

- A. Periductal stroma
- B. Interlobular stroma
- C. Intratumoral compartment
- D. Peritumoral compartment
- E. Subareolar area

Answer: **D. Peritumoral compartment**

Comment: Lymphovascular invasion is ideally evaluated in the peritumoral (tumor edge/periphery of invasive cancer) tissue due to the several pitfalls within the tumor that may mimic vascular invasion. Of these the artifactual tissue retraction is most important and most problematic. Therefore most authors agreed to evaluate lymphovascular invasion (predominantly lymphatic vessels) at the tumor periphery.

Q.54 The diagnosis of microinvasive breast carcinoma is made if the invasive tumor measures:

- A. 2 mm
- B. 5 mm
- C. 1 mm
- D. 0.5 mm
- E. 0.2 mm

Answer: C. 1 mm

Comment: By definition, **microinvasive carcinomas** are characterized by the extension of tumor cells beyond the basement membrane into the stroma with no focus exceeding 1 mm/0.1 cm in its largest dimension. Although, the cut-off may be subjective, one should render the diagnosis of microinvasive carcinoma only if one (or more) foci of unequivocal invasion into the stroma are present. The pathologist should also quantify the number of foci (if more than one is present) including the size of the largest focus. Microinvasive carcinoma is commonly seen in association with extensive high-grade ductal carcinoma in situ (DCIS).

Q.55 Macroscopic size of the breast cancer of 9 mm is categorized by AJCC TNM system as:

- A. pT1mi
- B. pT1a
- C. pT1b
- D. pT1c
- E. pT2

Answer: C. pT1b

Comment: American Joint Commission on Cancer System (AJCC) for the staging of tumor size (7th edition, revised in 2010) is routinely provided for all breast cancers (in situ and invasive). According to AJCC TNM, the tumor >5 mm and ≤10 mm are categorized as pT1b; the tumors ≥10 and ≤20 mm as pT1c category while tumors measuring ≥20 mm as pT2; pT1mi denotes microinvasive breast carcinoma (invasion ≤1 mm in its greatest dimension). The remaining pT1a category includes the invasive cancers between 1–5 mm.

Q.56 For early breast cancer surgical margins are considered clean if no tumor cells were observed:

- A. 1 mm from the ink
- B. 2 mm from the ink
- C. 5 mm from the ink
- D. No visible tumor cells on the ink
- E. 10 mm from the ink

Answer: D. No visible tumor cells on the ink

Comment: The surgical margins have been a matter of discussion for a long time. Recently, American Society of Clinical Oncology Endorsement of the Society of Surgical Oncology/American Society for Radiation Oncology Consensus Guideline have proposed a guideline for the assessment of margins for stage I and stage II breast cancer treated by breast-conserving surgery and radiotherapy (*Source:* Bucholz TA, et al. J Clin Oncol. 2014). According to this guideline, the margins are considered clean if no tumor cells are present at any inked margin.

Q.57 Axillary lymph node metastatic deposit measuring 3 mm is categorized as:

- A. Macrometastasis
- B. Micrometastasis
- C. Isolated tumor cells
- D. Occult metastasis

Answer: A. Macrometastasis

Comment: The status of axillary lymph nodes is still the single most important prognosticator for patients with invasive breast carcinomas. A metastatic deposit > 2 mm is defined as **macrometastasis** while the deposit between 0.2–2 mm (or more than 200 tumor cells) is called micrometastasis. Isolated tumor cells denote the tumor burden <0.2 mm (or less than 200 tumor cells). Micrometastases and isolated tumor cells are commonly called "occult metastases" and several recent studies indicated that their clinical relevance and impact on the patients' outcome are not significant.

Q.58 Sentinel lymph nodes should be sectioned at what thickness?

    A. 1 mm intervals
    B. 2 mm intervals
    C. 4 mm intervals
    D. 5 mm intervals

Answer: **B. 2 mm intervals**

Comment: Sentinel lymph node evaluation is a standard pathology practice for the patients with invasive breast cancer and extensive DCIS. The aim of sentinel lymph node cutting is to detect macrometastases (≥2 mm) and therefore lymph nodes are recommended to be cut at 2 mm thickness.

Q.59 Chemotherapeutic effects on the tumor cells include all the cytologic changes below, *except*:

    A. Eosinophilic cytoplasm with prominent vacuolization
    B. Nucleomegalia
    C. Multinucleation and vesicular chromatin
    D. Prominent atypia (bizarre cells)
    E. Increased mitotic activity

Answer: **E. Increased mitotic activity**

Comment: **Neoadjuvant chemotherapy** is increasingly used for the treatment of breast cancer. Cytotoxic drugs affect the cytology of the tumor cells but mitotic activity is usually not markedly changed. Cytotoxic effects usually increase the cellular atypia and pleomorphism of the tumor cells may be more prominent in comparison with the cell appearance before treatment with chemotherapy. Overall, histologic grade is usually not affected by neoadjuvant chemotherapy.

Q.60 A core biopsy of the breast in a 63-year-old female with a previous history of radiotherapy for high-grade DCIS in the same breast is shown in Figure 6.9. What is the best diagnosis?

    A. Atypical ductal hyperplasia (ADH)
    B. Ductal carcinoma in situ (DCIS)
    C. Radiation-induced changes
    D. Usual ductal hyperplasia (UDH)

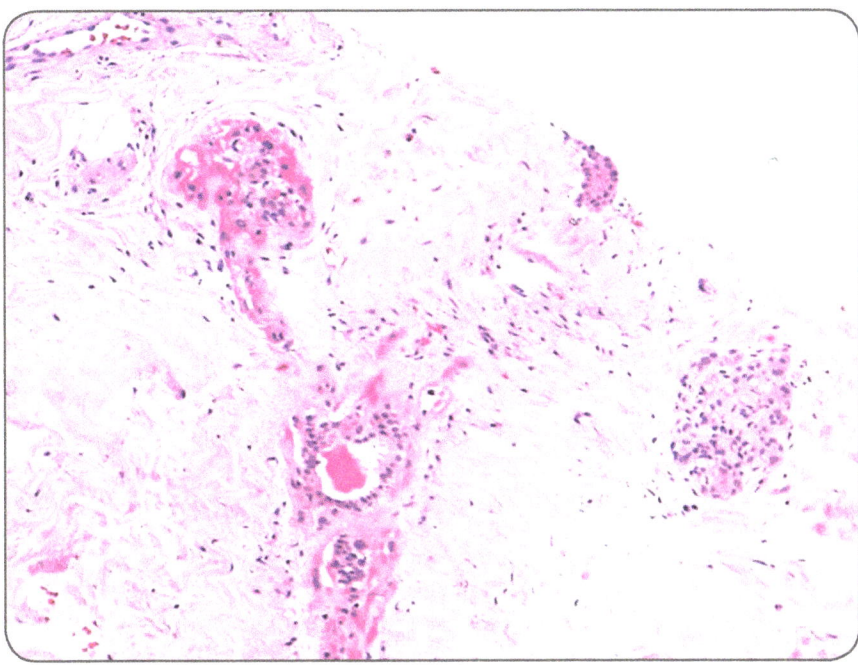

Figure 6.9

Answer: **C. Radiation-induced changes**

Comment: The figure shows scattered atypical cells in the terminal ductal lobular unit (TDLU). These alterations represent radiation-induced changes in the breast epithelium. The patient underwent breast-conserving surgery and radiation therapy for high-grade ductal carcinoma in situ. Note the lack of the extension of TDLU as well as other signs of atypical proliferation (increased cellularity, mitotic figures).

Q.61 What is the MD Anderson calculator used for?

- **A.** To predict response to chemotherapy
- **B.** To predict response to endocrine therapy
- **C.** To evaluate the amount of residual cancer after chemotherapy
- **D.** To predict survival

Answer: **C. To evaluate the amount of residual cancer after chemotherapy**

Comment: MD Anderson Residual Burden Calculator (RCB) has been developed as a tool to quantify the tumor response to the neoadjuvant chemotherapy [range: from pCR (pathologic complete response) to chemoresistant tumors]. Its calculation includes both the primary cancer (its size, microscopic cellularity, presence of in situ component), and axillary lymph nodes [number and size of metastatic lymph node(s)].

Q.62 Complete pathologic response (pCR) following neoadjuvant chemotherapy is obtained in approximately how many cases?

   A. ~20%
   B. ~50%
   C. 5%
   D. 70%
   E. 80%

Answer: A. ~20%

Comment: pCR, defined as no residual invasive cancer following chemotherapy, is seen in 10–30% of all breast carcinomas. The majority of breast cancers (~70%) have a partial response while 10–15% of breast carcinomas are completely chemoresistant. The best chemotherapy response is observed in Her2-positive and triple-negative breast carcinomas while luminal breast cancers exhibit a poor response to chemotherapy (particularly if proliferation index is low).

Q.63 According to the ASCO/CAP guideline (2010), the tumor is considered estrogen receptor (ER) positive if at least:

   A. 5% of tumor cells show nuclear staining
   B. 1% of tumor cells show nuclear staining
   C. 10% of tumor cells show nuclear staining
   D. 20% of tumor cells show nuclear staining

Answer: B. 1% of tumor cells

Comment: The most recent ASCO/CAP guideline (2010) defined the invasive breast carcinomas to be positive for ER if at least 1% of tumor cells show nuclear staining. The pathologist should also report the intensity of the staining (strong, medium, weak), when combined with percentage may give a score (e.g. Allred score). For all IHC assays for ER and PR it is critically important to include adequate internal positive controls to avoid false-negative results, which still may be seen in up to 20% of tested cases. ER is also routinely evaluated on all cases of DCIS.

Q.64 Which of the following biomarkers is routinely utilized for proliferation rate assessment in breast cancer?

   A. Ki-67
   B. Topoisomerase II
   C. Proliferating cell nuclear antigen (PCNA)
   D. Topoisomerase I
   E. Phosphohistone H3

Answer: A. Ki-67

Comment: Ki-67 using MIB-1 antibody is usually employed for proliferation assessment in breast cancer and recommended by the St Gallen Consensus Conference. The threshold for estimation has been controversial with a lot of debate in the published literature. Still, it can be useful in the assessment and discrimination of luminal breast tumors (Luminal A vs. Luminal B) while it has a little or no utility in the proliferation assessment of highly proliferating breast cancers such as Her2-positive and triple-negative breast cancers. All other biomarkers also stain neoplastic cells in various phases of proliferation but none of them is routinely employed and validated.

Q.65 What is the score for Her2 expression in the breast carcinoma shown in the Figure 6.10?

A. Score 1+
B. Score 2+
C. Score 3+
D. Score 0
E. Non-interpretative

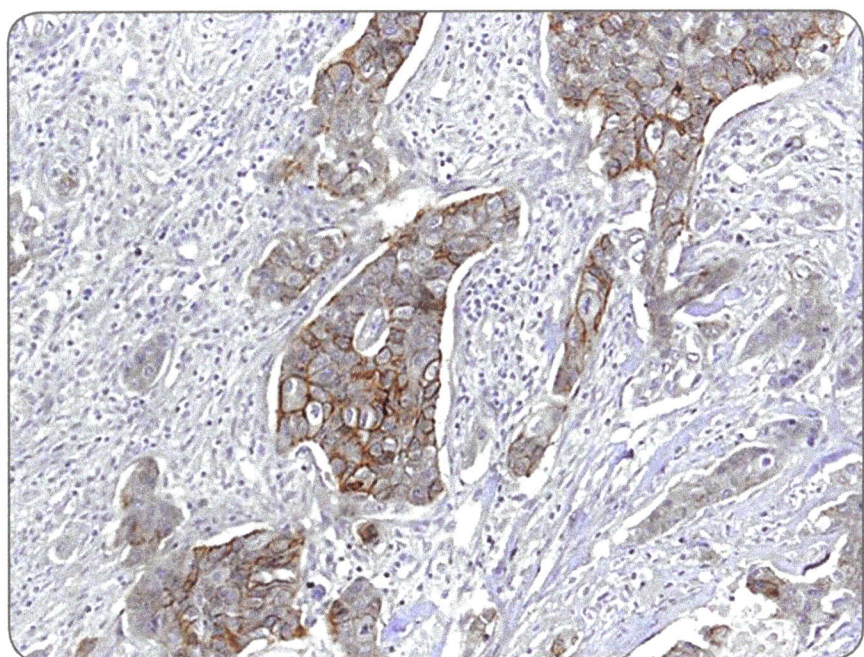

Figure 6.10

Answer: **B. Score 2+**

Comment: The present slide shows incomplete, weak to moderate Her2 expression in more than 10% of the tumor cells, consistent with Her2 borderline (score 2+) expression. This pattern requires additional evaluation by in-situ hybridization assays (e.g. FISH or CISH) to explore the amplification of *Her2/neu* gene. Note the lack of Her2 expression in adjacent stromal cells.

Q.66 What is the most appropriate immunohistochemical marker for identifying angiolymphatic invasion in breast cancer?

A. CD31
B. CD34
C. Factor VIII-related antigen
D. D2-40 (podoplanin)
E. CD105 (endoglin)

Answer: **D. D2-40 (podoplanin)**

Comment: **D2-40 (podoplanin)** is a specific marker for endothelium of lymphatic vessels while all other markers stain endothelium of blood vessels. Given that lymphatic invasion is the most common in breast cancer, D2-40 is the most suitable marker for **lymphovascular invasion** in breast cancer. CD105 (endoglin) is a selective marker of neoangiogenesis while CD31, CD34 and Factor VIII-related antigen stain all blood vessels.

Q.67 Which of the following molecular subtypes of breast cancer is poorly characterized?

 A. Basal-like breast cancer subtype
 B. Normal breast-like subtype
 C. Luminal subtypes (A and B)
 D. Her2 subtype

Answer: B. Normal breast-like subtype

Comment: Although initially described as a distinct molecular subtype of breast cancer, normal breast-like subtype has not been confirmed in subsequent studies. It remained a poorly characterized and according to some authors this subtype represents an artifact caused by the contamination of tumor samples by normal breast tissue. In contrast, luminal A and B tumor, Her2 and basal-like breast tumors have been widely characterized although a full clinical value of these subtypes has not been established yet.

Q.68 Which of the following subtypes of breast cancer is a prototype of invasive breast carcinoma with mixed features (ductal and lobular)?

 A. Tubulolobular carcinoma
 B. Invasive cribriform carcinoma
 C. Pleomorphic lobular carcinoma
 D. Pleomorphic carcinoma

Answer: A. Tubulolobular carcinoma

Comment: **Tubulolobular carcinoma** of the breast is rare variant of mammary carcinoma sharing the features of both ductal (in a form of tubules) and lobular breast carcinoma. It has been traditionally considered as a variant of lobular carcinoma although it typically exhibits positivity for E-cadherin. Invasive cribriform carcinoma is a low-grade, special type of breast cancer, composed predominantly (>90%) of cribriform structures. Pleomorphic lobular carcinoma is a high-grade variant of invasive lobular carcinoma while pleomorphic carcinoma is a rare variant of high-grade invasive ductal carcinoma with prominent nuclear atypia and bizarre giant tumor cells.

Q.69 All of the below listed special types of breast carcinoma are associated with a favorable clinical outcome, *except*:

 A. Tubular carcinoma
 B. Cribriform carcinoma
 C. Adenoid cystic carcinoma
 D. Pure mucinous carcinoma
 E. Apocrine carcinoma

Answer: E. Apocrine carcinoma

Comment: Tubular, cribriform and mucinous carcinomas are typically low-grade carcinomas, ER-positive, Her2 negative carcinomas with a low proliferation rate ("Luminal-A tumors") associated with an excellent prognosis and outcome. Adenoid cystic carcinomas (ACC) although exhibiting a triple-negative immunophenotype (ER-/PR-/Her2-) have a similar clinical behavior. The clinical outcome of the patients with apocrine carcinoma has been a subject of debate with contradictory results in the published literature. However, most studies showed that patients with apocrine carcinoma have a similar prognosis as patients with ductal carcinoma of no-special-type when appropriately matched.

Q.70 What is the threshold for a certain morphologic subtype of breast cancer to be defined as special type?

- A. >50%
- B. >75%
- C. 50–75%
- D. >90%
- E. 100%

Answer: D. >90%

Comment: Special types of breast carcinomas are defined as breast carcinomas with a specific morphology present in >90% of the specimen (e.g. micropapillary, tubular, mucinous, apocrine, papillary). Some of the special types also have distinct molecular genetic and clinical characteristics (e.g. lobular carcinoma, adenoid cystic carcinoma, medullary carcinoma).

Q.71 What is the best diagnosis for the breast tumor shown in Figure 6.11?

- A. Apocrine carcinoma
- B. Medullary carcinoma
- C. Metaplastic carcinoma
- D. Glycogen-rich carcinoma
- E. Solid papillary carcinoma

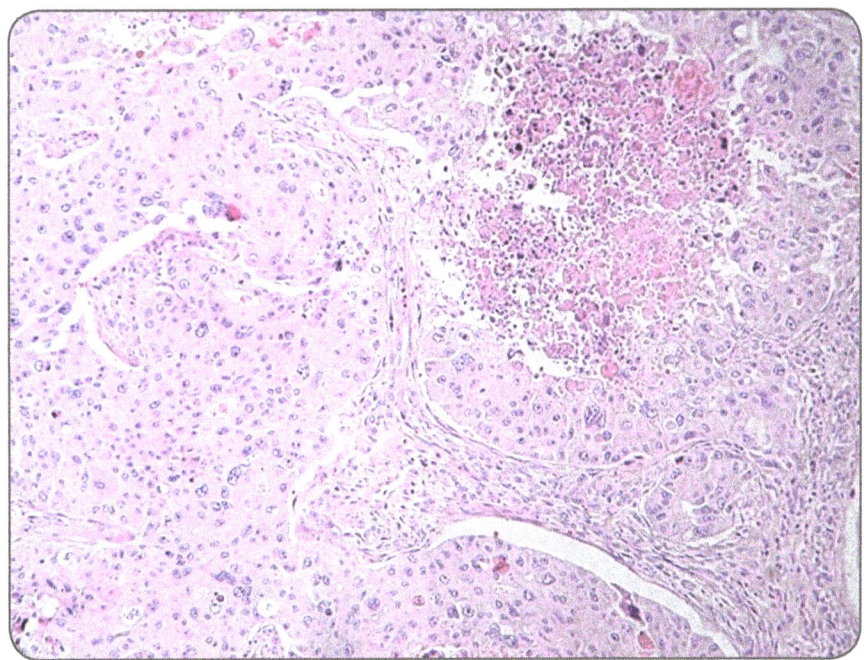

Figure 6.11

Answer: C. Metaplastic carcinoma

Comment: Morphological characteristics of the tumor are consistent with metaplastic carcinoma (squamous differentiation, high-grade variant). It is morphologically heterogeneous group of breast tumors, which includes squamous cell carcinoma, metaplastic carcinoma with mesenchymal differentiation, low-grade adenosquamous carcinoma, spindle cell carcinoma, and fibromatosis-like carcinoma (the 2011 WHO Breast Working Group). Of note, foci of squamous differentiation may be seen in other breast carcinoma subtypes including ductal of no-special-type and medullary carcinoma. Pure squamous cell carcinomas in the breast are rare.

Q.72 Figure 6.12 shows a biopsy specimen of the nipple/areola complex from a 54-year-old female. What is the best diagnosis?

   A. Malignant melanoma
   B. Erosive adenomatosis of the nipple
   C. Squamous cell carcinoma in situ (Bowen disease)
   D. Paget disease of the nipple
   E. Toker cell hyperplasia

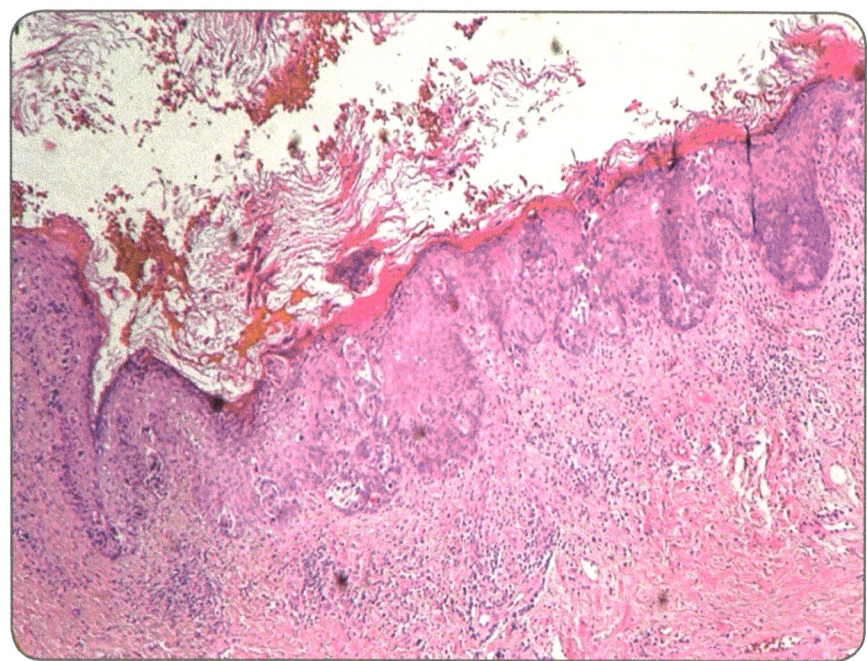

Figure 6.12

Answer: D. Paget disease of the nipple

Comment: Hematoxylin and eosin figure shows infiltration of the nipple epidermis with large, high-grade malignant cells. **Paget disease** is commonly associated with underlying high-grade DCIS or invasive carcinoma (>95% cases) and is typically positive for CK7 and EMA (not shown). Her2/neu overexpression is also commonly present (~50%). Malignant melanoma is rare in the nipple epidermis and is typically S-100 positive and negative for epithelial markers. **Erosive adenomatosis** (florid papillomatosis of the nipple/nipple adenoma) is a well-known clinical mimicker of Paget disease, but microscopic features are different (benign tumor; relatively circumscribed glandular proliferation that may involve the nipple epidermis). Bowen disease (squamous cell carcinoma in situ) affecting the nipple epidermis is also an uncommon lesion. Benign intraepidermal cells with cytoplasmic clearing that represent either keratinocytes or **Toker cells** may also be confused for the Paget cells.

Q.73 All the statements regarding invasive lobular carcinoma are correct, *except*:

   A. Constitutes ~10% of all breast carcinomas
   B. Frequently multifocal and bilateral
   C. Associated with LCIS in ~80% of the cases
   D. Has a characteristic mammographic appearance
   E. Has characteristic cytologic features

Answer: D. Characteristic mammographic appearance

Comment: Invasive lobular carcinomas have distinct cytologic features, but radiologically it may have indistinguishable features from invasive ductal carcinoma. However, lobular carcinomas may have subtle mammographic appearance presenting as either asymmetric density of architectural distortion of breast parenchyma. In such cases, magnetic resonance imaging (MRI) may be helpful in the proper estimation and evaluation of the lesion extent.

Q.74 Medullary carcinomas of the breast are characterized by all the following microscopic attributes, *except:*

- A. Syncytial growth pattern >50% of the tumor
- B. Dense lymphoplasmacytic infiltration
- C. Circumscription
- D. High nuclear grade
- E. No glandular differentiation

Answer: **A. Syncytial growth pattern >50% of the tumor**

Comment: **Syncytial growth pattern** in >75% of the tumor is required for medullary carcinoma. This strict classification has substantially improved the interobserver variability among pathologists and reduced the incidence of "pure" **medullary carcinomas** below 1%. Breast cancers that fulfill some but not all the above criteria are usually called either "atypical medullary carcinomas" or "invasive carcinomas with medullary features".

Q.75 Which of the following subtypes of breast cancer shows grossly circumscribed appearance?

- A. Invasive ductal carcinoma (NOS)
- B. Invasive lobular carcinoma
- C. Medullary carcinoma
- D. Adenoid cystic carcinoma
- E. Micropapillary carcinoma

Answer: **C. Medullary carcinoma**

Comment: **Medullary carcinoma** has typically a well-circumscribed gross appearance followed by the microscopic circumscribed growth. Other subtypes usually present as a firm, infiltrative mass with stellate or spiculated contours. Invasive lobular carcinoma may even present without grossly evident mass with the presence of tumor cells only on microscopic examination.

Q.76 Which of the following subtypes of invasive lobular carcinoma is associated with a more aggressive clinical course and poor outcome?

- A. Pleomorphic variant
- B. Alveolar variant
- C. Solid variant
- D. Trabecular variant
- E. Classical variant

Answer: **A. Pleomorphic variant**

Comment: **Pleomorphic variant of lobular carcinoma** appears to behave analogue to the invasive ductal carcinoma grade 3. This subtype is frequently ER and PR positive, but also may be Her2/neu positive with underlying *Her2/neu* gene amplification. Other subtypes of lobular carcinoma are typically of lower histologic grade (grade 1 or 2), steroid receptor (ER and PR) positive, but Her2/neu negative. Of note, a subset of pleomorphic lobular carcinomas may overlap with apocrine carcinomas at both morphologic and molecular level.

Q.77 Core biopsy of the mass in a 55-year-old female with a previous history of ipsilateral LCIS and contralateral invasive ductal carcinoma is shown in Figure 6.13. What is the best diagnosis?

A. Florid ductal hyperplasia and invasive ductal carcinoma
B. Lobular neoplasia and malignant cells within the angiolymphatic spaces
C. Atypical ductal hyperplasia
D. Neuroendocrine carcinoma

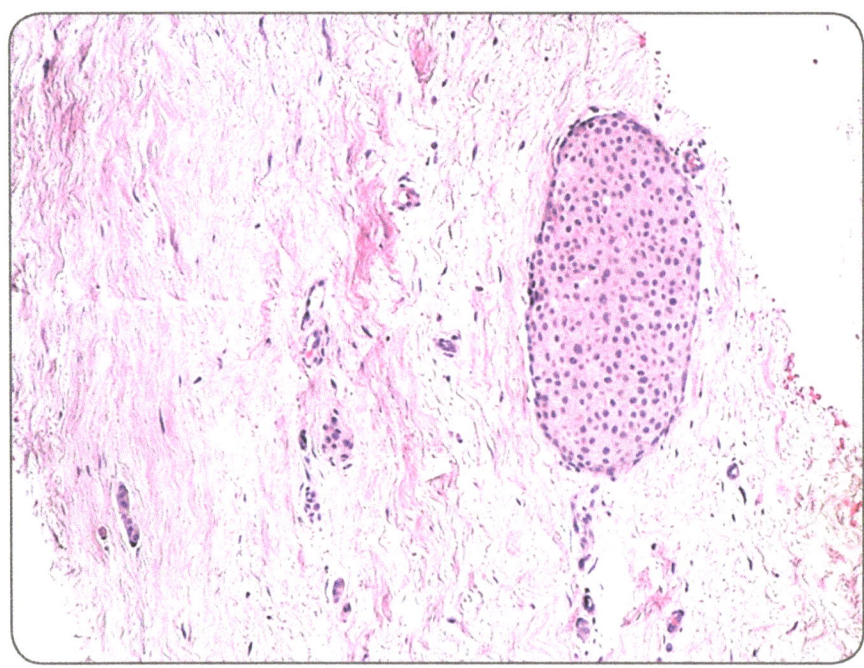

Figure 6.13

Answer: **B. Lobular neoplasia and malignant cells within the angiolymphatic spaces**

Comment: In the left part of the figure emboli of neoplastic cells are easily visible within the **angiolymphatic spaces**. Focus on the right side represents a **lobular neoplasia** [note the presence of basal/myoepithelial cells (darker cells) that are not present in case of neuroendocrine carcinoma].

Q.78 A characteristic "peau d'orange" appearance of inflammatory carcinoma of the breast includes all, *except*:

A. Skin erythema
B. Edema
C. Pigmentation
D. Induration
E. Tenderness

Answer: **C. Pigmentation**

Comment: **Inflammatory carcinoma** is a rare subtype of breast carcinoma with an aggressive clinical course. It presents with the tumor emboli within the dermal lymphatics resulting in a characteristic skin appearance (erythema, edema, induration and tenderness), but pigmentation is not seen. It is believed that the "peau d'orange" is a consequence of the lymphatic obstruction. Inflammatory carcinoma cells are ER and PR positive in ~50% of the cases while *Her2/neu* gene amplification is present in approximately 40% of the cases.

Q.79 Which subtype of breast cancer shows most often neuroendocrine differentiation?
- A. Lipid-rich
- B. Apocrine
- C. Mucinous (hypercellular variant)
- D. Mucinous (paucicellular variant)
- E. Polymorphous carcinoma

Answer: **C. Mucinous (hypercellular variant)**

Comment: Neuroendocrine differentiation may be seen (up to 30%) in various breast carcinoma subtypes including ductal carcinoma of no-special-type as well as in some special types, particularly in hypercellular variant of mucinous carcinomas and solid papillary carcinomas. Other above mentioned subtypes rarely exhibit neuroendocrine differentiation.

Q.80 Carcinomas with neuroendocrine differentiation belong to the following molecular cluster of breast carcinomas:
- A. Luminal A
- B. Luminal B
- C. Triple-negative
- D. Her2 positive

Answer: **A. Luminal A**

Comment: Neuroendocrine carcinomas are typically ER and PR positive while Her2 overexpression is absent, thus clustering within the luminal A subgroup. More than 50% of high-grade (small cell) neuroendocrine carcinomas also express both steroid receptors. Similar molecular profiles have other breast carcinomas with neuroendocrine differentiation (mucinous and solid papillary carcinomas).

Q.81 What is the best diagnosis for the malignant breast tumor shown in Figure 6.14?
- A. Classical lobular carcinoma
- B. Pleomorphic lobular carcinoma
- C. Apocrine carcinoma
- D. Malignant lymphoma

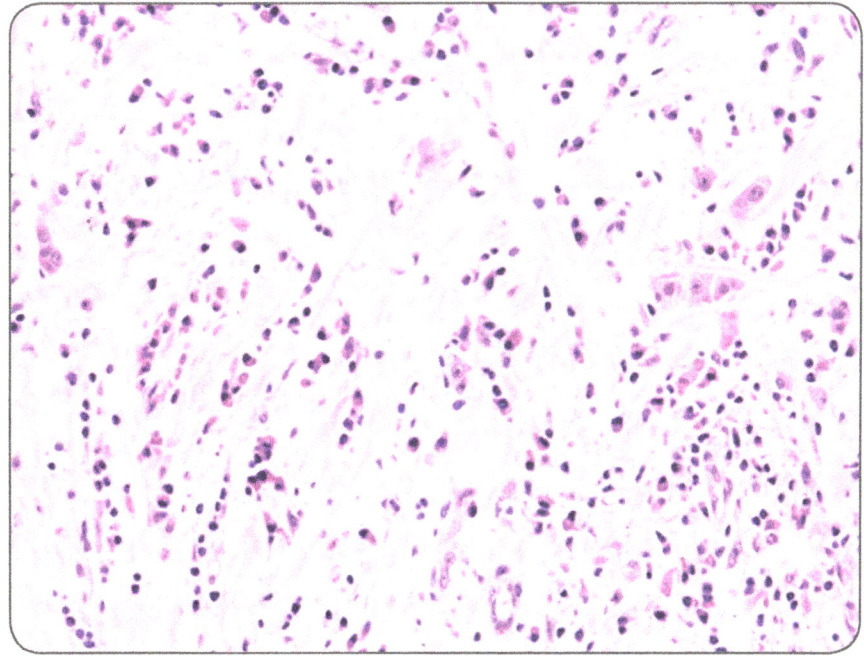

Figure 6.14

Answer: B. Pleomorphic lobular carcinoma

Comment: Figure 6.14 shows an invasive mammary carcinoma composed of single and sheets of moderately to highly atypical, discohesive cells with abundant eosinophilic cytoplasm. All these findings are consistent with **pleomorphic lobular carcinoma**. In contrast to classical lobular carcinoma, atypia of the tumor cells is marked while discohesiveness followed by the loss of E-cadherin discriminates it from apocrine carcinoma.

Q.82 What is the best diagnosis for the malignant breast tumor shown in Figure 6.15?

    A. Invasive cribriform carcinoma
    B. Ductal carcinoma in situ (DCIS)
    C. Adenoid cystic carcinoma
    D. Medullary carcinoma
    E. Lobular carcinoma in situ

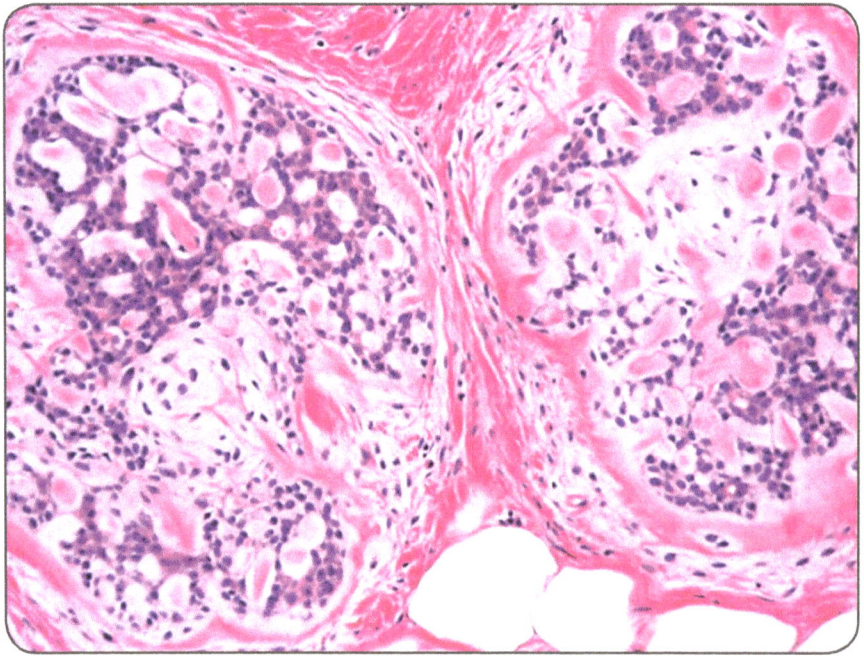

Figure 6.15

Answer: C. Adenoid cystic carcinoma

Comment: The microphotographs shows the tumor composed of cribriform and tubular formations with eosinophilic hyaline material within the lumen. The tumor is composed of a dual-cell population of luminal and myoepithelial/basal cells, both of which may be readily distinguished by immunohistochemistry. Adenoid cystic carcinoma (ACC) exhibits a triple-negative phenotype (ER-/PR-/Her2-), but is associated with an indolent clinical course and excellent outcome.

Q.83 Figure 6.16 shows cytokeratin 5/6 expression in an invasive breast cancer. What is the most likely diagnosis?

A. Ductal carcinoma in situ (DCIS)
B. Squamous cell carcinoma
C. Invasive ductal carcinoma with basal phenotype
D. Metastatic carcinoma
E. Metaplastic carcinoma

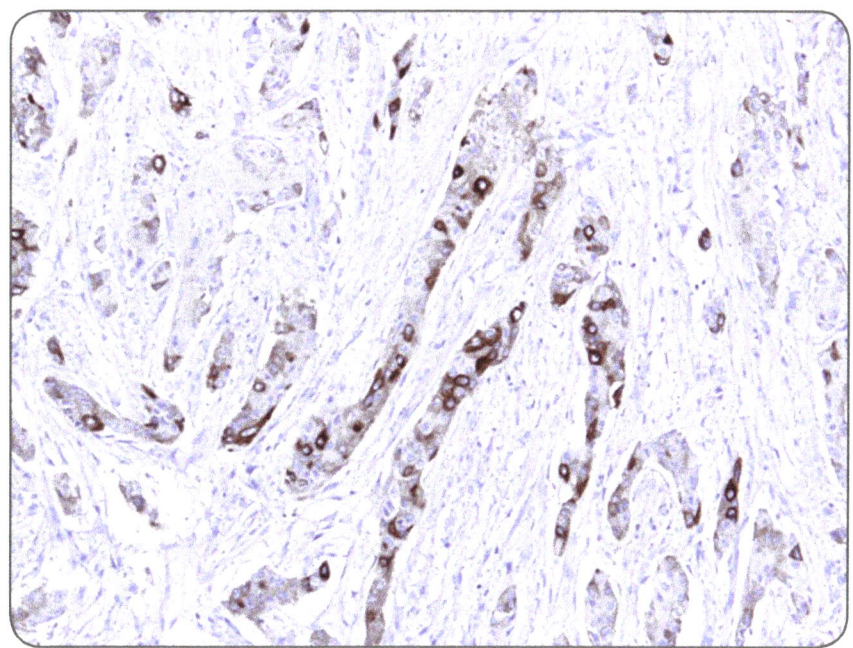

Figure 6.16

Answer: C. Invasive ductal carcinoma with basal phenotype

Comment: The photomicrograph shows invasive mammary carcinoma with ductal morphology that exhibits focal CK5/6 expression. CK5/6 is a sensitive marker of basal/myoepithelial cells in various tissues as well as stratified squamous epithelium. Expression of basal markers may be seen in a subset of invasive mammary carcinomas with triple-negative immunophenotype (ER-/PR-/Her2-) and basal features by gene expression profiling (so called "basal-like breast carcinomas"). Primary squamous cell carcinomas of the breast are very rare and belong to the category of metaplastic breast carcinomas. Their morphology may be similar to the squamous carcinomas arising elsewhere in the body. Metastatic carcinomas to the breast exhibiting CK5/6 positivity are very uncommon but clinical information/imaging may help rendering the correct diagnosis in the challenging cases.

Q.84 The specimen shown in Figure 6.17 was obtained from axilla of a woman known to have a breast tumor. What is the best diagnosis?

A. Micropapillary carcinoma
B. Metastatic carcinoma to the axilla with perineural invasion
C. Neuroendocrine carcinoma
D. Primary axillary carcinoma

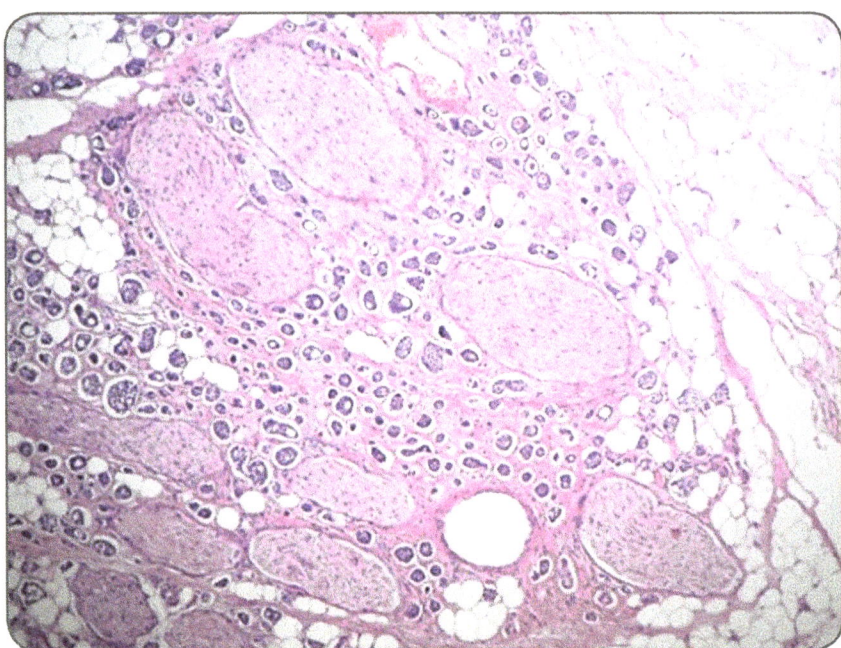

Figure 6.17

Answer: **B. Metastatic carcinoma to the axilla with perineural invasion.**

Comment: The Figure shows extensive infiltration of the axillary fatty tissue with metastatic breast carcinoma. Foci of perineural invasion are also readily identifiable. Perineural invasion is a commonly seen in breast cancer and indicates tumor aggressiveness. Of note, some metastatic breast carcinomas to the axilla may resemble micropapillary morphology that is characterized by the tumor clusters within the irregular empty "stromal" spaces (as seen here).

Q.85 Figure 6.18 shows a core biopsy from the rapidly growing breast mass in a 67-year-old woman. What is the best diagnosis?

    A. Medullary carcinoma
    B. Pleomorphic lobular carcinoma
    C. Pleomorphic carcinoma
    D. Carcinoma with osteoclast-like stromal giant cells
    E. Neuroendocrine carcinoma

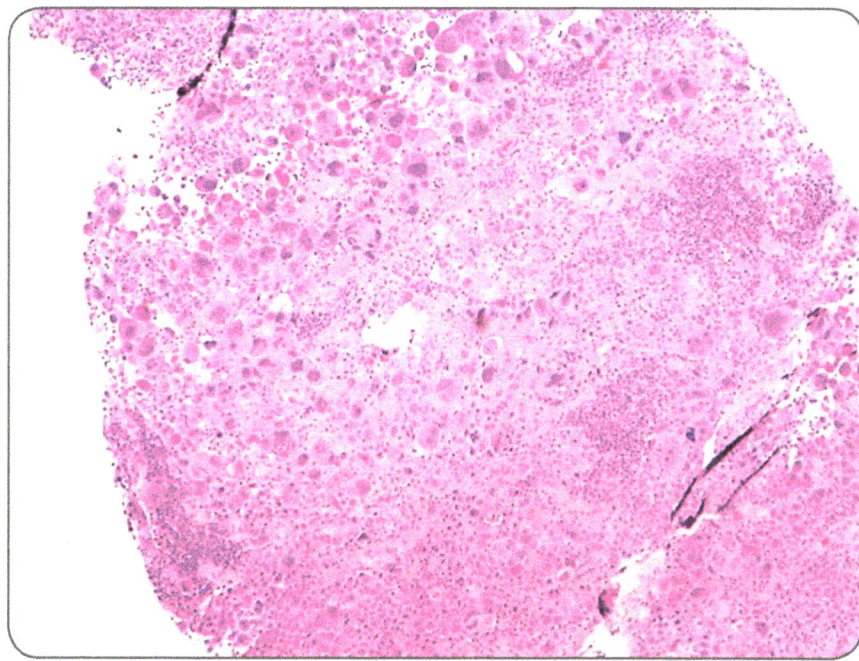

Figure 6.18

Answer: C. Pleomorphic carcinoma

Comment: The Figure shows an infiltrating breast cancer composed predominantly of highly pleomorphic, giant, and bizarre neoplastic cells with high mitotic activity. These cells were confirmed to be of epithelial origin (Cam5.2 and AE1/AE3 positive, not shown). In contrast, pleomorphic lobular carcinoma is composed of discohesive neoplastic cells while carcinoma with osteoclast-like giant stromal cells contains stromal cells (CD68 positive, cytokeratin negative) that accompany invasive ductal carcinoma. Stromal cells also lack mitotic activity. Medullary carcinoma is also composed of atypical epithelial cells with marked pleomorphism, but giant and bizarre neoplastic cells are not seen.

Q.86 Figure 6.19 shows a core biopsy of an invasive breast carcinoma diagnosed in a 70-year-old woman. What is the best diagnosis?

A. Carcinoma with metaplastic features
B. Carcinoma with medullary features
C. Carcinoma with osteoclast-like stromal giant cells
D. Carcinoma with choriocarcinomatous features

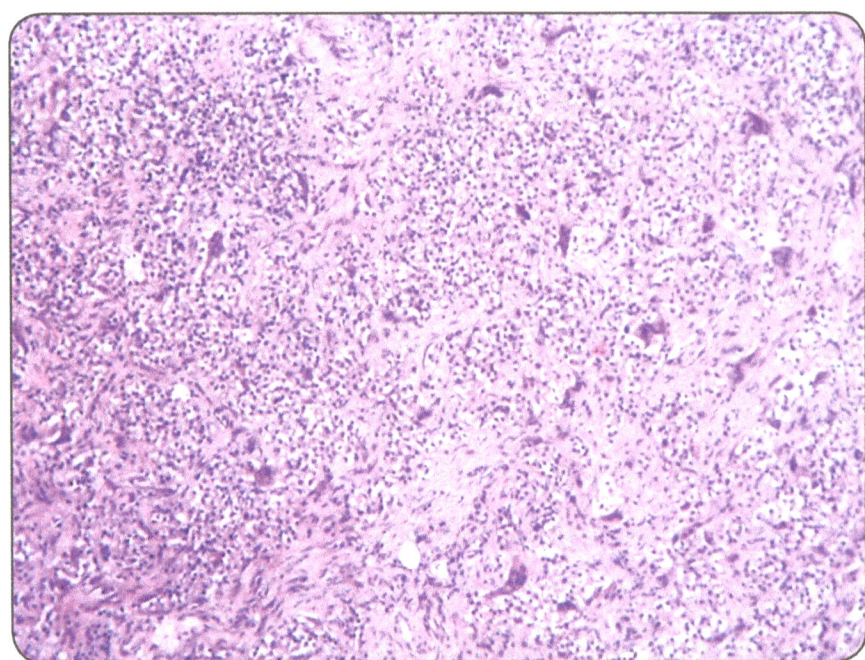

Figure 6.19

Answer: C. Carcinoma with osteoclast-like stromal giant cells

Comment: The Figure shows moderately differentiated invasive ductal carcinoma with **osteoclast-like giant stromal cells**. This is a rare subtype of breast cancer. The presence of stromal cells appears not to affect the patient's prognosis that is related to the features of the associated tumor cells. The stromal cells are positive for histiocytic markers (e.g. CD68) and negative for epithelial markers (cytokeratins and EMA) and S-100.

Q.87 WHO Working Group proposed in 2011 the diagnostic criteria for distinguishing between benign, borderline and malignant phyllodes tumors. These include all, *except:*
  A. Tumor borders
  B. Stromal cellularity/atypia
  C. Mitotic activity
  D. Cleft-like spaces
  E. Stromal overgrowth

Answer: D. Cleft-like spaces

Comment: Cleft-like, epithelial-lined spaces with "leaf-like" projections that are surrounded by the dense stromal proliferation favor the diagnosis of phyllodes tumor over cellular fibroadenomas; however, cleft-like spaces are not reliable for the estimation and distinction between benign, borderline and malignant phyllodes tumors. Along with the four above mentioned characteristics, the presence of malignant heterologous elements (bone, cartilage) strongly favors the diagnosis of malignant phyllodes tumor, even if other features (criteria) are absent. Benign heterologous elements (bone, cartilage, adipose tissue, skeletal muscle) may be seen not only in benign phyllodes tumors, but also in fibroadenomas.

Q.88 Figure 6.20 shows a breast tumor removed from a 45 year-old woman. What is the best diagnosis?

A. Periductal stromal sarcoma
B. Benign phyllodes tumor
C. Complex fibroadenoma
D. Malignant phyllodes tumor
E. Metaplastic carcinoma

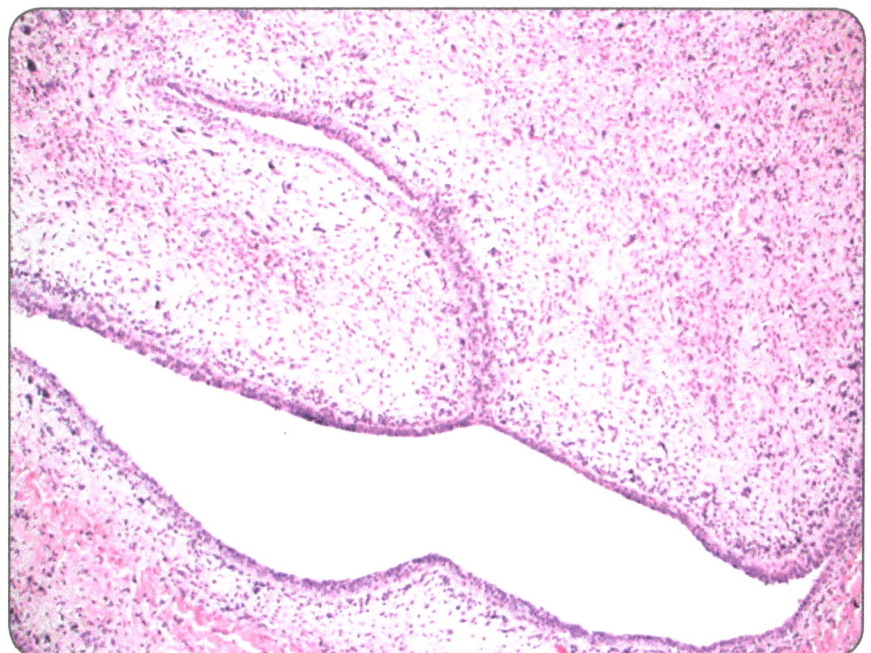

Figure 6.20

Answer: D. Malignant phyllodes tumor

Comment: Figure 6.20 shows a biphasic, fibroepithelial tumor with "leaf-like" processes and highly cellular stromal component with prominent atypia suggestive of malignant phyllodes tumor. In contrast, fibroadenomas lack prominent stromal proliferation, which may be seen in metaplastic carcinomas (spindle cell variant) but the stromal cells are positive for epithelial markers (e.g. wide-spectrum keratins [AE1/AE3, Cam5.2, MNF116]; of note expression of epithelial markers may be focal and weak). Also, metaplastic carcinomas are rarely biphasic. Periductal stromal sarcoma is a rare breast malignancy that lacks "leaf-like" processes with spindle cell proliferation around open tubules. However, the progression from periductal stromal sarcoma to phyllodes tumor has been described.

Q.89 Which of the following breast tumors is considered to be derived from the skin?

A. Dermatofibrosarcoma protuberans
B. Angiosarcoma
C. Liposarcoma
D. Leiomyosarcoma
E. Osteosarcoma

Answer: A. Dermatofibrosarcoma protuberans

Comment: Primary sarcomas of the breast apart from angiosarcomas are very rare. In contrast to other rare soft tissue tumors listed above, **dermatofibrosarcoma protuberans** typically affects skin, not breast parenchyma.

Q.90 Which of the following is the most common primary sarcoma of the breast?
- A. Periductal stromal sarcoma
- B. Angiosarcoma
- C. Liposarcoma
- D. Fibrosarcoma
- E. Pseudoangiomatous stromal hyperplasia (PASH)

Answer: B. Angiosarcoma

Comment: **Angiosarcoma** is the most common primary sarcoma of the breast (~0.05% of all breast malignancies). It can arise spontaneously (primary) or more frequently following radiotherapy of the breast (secondary angiosarcoma). Periductal stromal sarcoma is a rare, biphasic neoplasm characterized by the atypical stromal proliferation around benign epithelium of the breast; PASH is benign myofibroblastic proliferation that may mimic a vascular lesion. Primary lipo- and fibrosarcomas are very rare in the breast-like all other sarcomas (leiomyosarcoma, rhabdomyosarcoma, malignant peripheral nerve sheath tumor). One should also consider metastatic sarcomas in differential diagnosis when diagnosing soft tissue lesion in the breast. Noteworthy, a broad IHC panel (broad spectrum cytokeratins, e.g. Cam5.2, AE1/AE3, MNF116, CK5/6, p63) should always be employed to rule out the metaplastic (spindle cell) carcinoma or malignant phyllodes tumor with stromal overgrowth (the presence of cleft-like spaces is a clue).

Q.91 Which of the following is the most common metastatic neoplasms to the breast?
- A. Sarcomas
- B. Gynecological cancers
- C. Lymphomas
- D. Gastric cancer
- E. Lung cancer

Answer: C. Lymphomas

Comment: **Metastatic tumors** to the breast are uncommon, constituting <1% of all breast cancers. Malignant lymphomas (predominantly non-Hodgkin lymphomas) are the most common secondary malignancies in the breast. Various carcinomas and sarcoma rarely metastasize to the breast.

Q.92 What is the most common subtype of primary lymphoma arising in the breast?
- A. MALT lymphoma
- B. Diffuse large B-cell lymphoma
- C. Hodgkin lymphoma
- D. Follicular lymphoma
- E. Anaplastic large cell lymphoma

Answer: B. Diffuse large B-cell lymphoma

Comment: **Lymphomas** affecting the breast (either primary or secondary) are very rare, constituting <1% of all breast malignancies. They are more frequently secondary due to the disseminated lymphoma arising elsewhere in the body. Nearly all primary breast lymphomas (defined as tumors limited to the breast and axillary lymph nodes in patients without previous history of lymphoproliferative disease) are non-Hodgkin lymphomas whereas Hodgkin lymphoma is exceedingly rare. Diffuse large B-cell lymphoma is the most common lymphoma affecting the breast while all other subtypes are uncommon.

Q.93 Figure 6.21 shows the core biopsy of the tumor mass diagnosed in a 50-year-old woman. The tumor cells were diffusely positive for WT-1 and negative for GCDFP-15. What is the most likely diagnosis?

   A. Invasive ductal carcinoma
   B. Invasive papillary carcinoma of the breast
   C. Micropapillary carcinoma of the breast
   D. Metastatic serous carcinoma

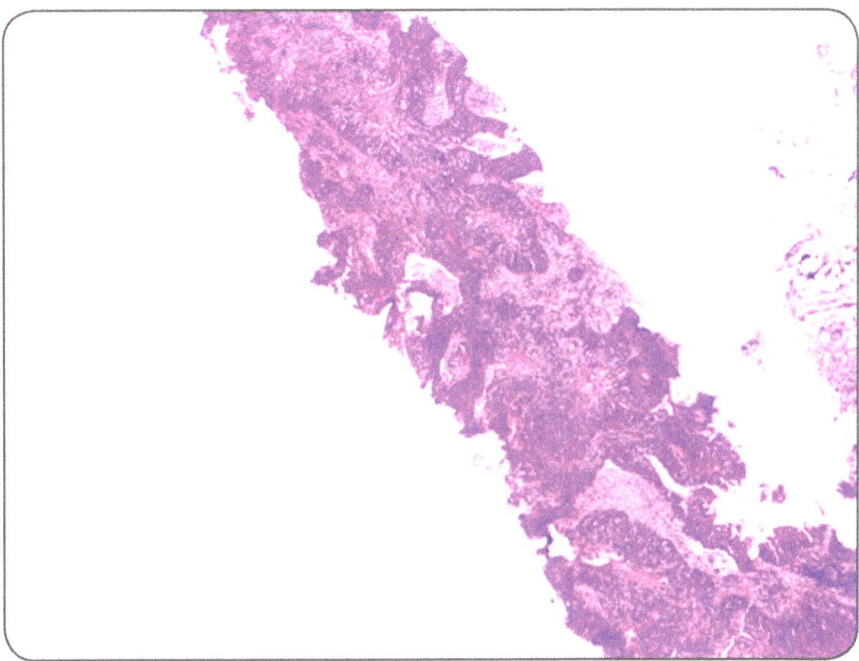

Figure 6.21

Answer: **D. Metastatic serous carcinoma**

Comment: The morphology indicates a high-grade carcinoma with papillary architecture that may overlap with primary, high-grade breast carcinomas with similar morphology. However, GCDFP-15 negativity along with diffuse and strong WT-1 positivity and clinical information on advanced (bulky) peritoneal disease were consistent with **metastatic** high-grade serous carcinoma of the peritoneum. Of note, some breast carcinomas (e.g. micropapillary carcinoma) may be occasionally positive for WT-1 but the presented case lacked the typical morphologic characteristics of primary micropapillary carcinoma of the breast.

Q.94 What is the most common lesion of the male breast?

   A. Intraductal papilloma
   B. Fibroadenoma
   C. Carcinoma NOS
   D. Gynecomastia
   E. DCIS

Answer: **D. Gynecomastia**

Comment: **Gynecomastia** is the most common lesion in male breast. Its etiology remains largely unknown although it may be associated with endocrine disorders (increased estrogen, decreased androgen) and some drugs (e.g. digitalis, antidepressants). Invasive **ductal carcinoma** and **DCIS** are uncommon although their frequency may be increased among men with Klinefelter syndrome and some hereditary cancer syndromes (e.g. *BRCA2* syndrome). **Fibroadenoma** and intraductal papilloma are very rare in the male breast.

CHAPTER 7

Immunohistochemistry and Genetics

Q.1 Which of the following anti-cytokeratin antibodies is best for identifying the lesion shown in Figure 7.1 as extramammary Paget disease of the vulva?

    A. anti-CK1
    B. anti-CK5
    C. anti-CK7
    D. anti-CK19
    E. anti-CK20

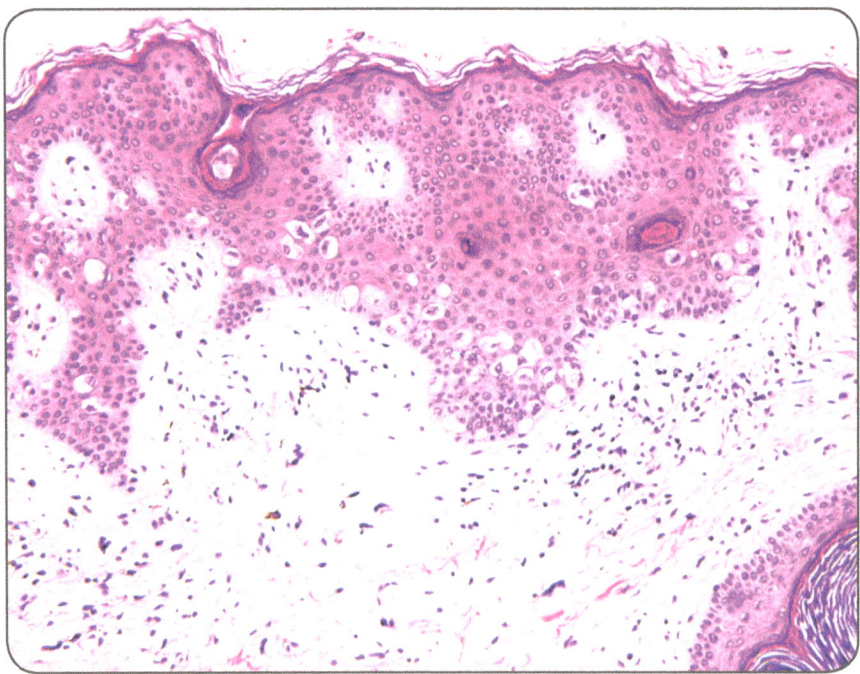

Figure 7.1

Answer: C. anti-CK7

Comment: **Vulvar extramammary Paget disease** is an intraepithelial carcinoma. Tumor cells infiltrating the epidermis react with antibodies to **CK7**. Antibody to CK7 does not react with normal vulvar epidermis and thus it is easy to recognize the CK7 positive neoplastic cells. Since, the monoclonal antibody **CAM5.2** recognizes both CK7 and CK8, it can be also used.

Contd...

Contd...

The cell of origin of vulvar Paget disease is not known, but most authorities believe that the tumors originate from Toker cells in the neck of breast-like glands found in this anatomic location. Toker cells are also CK7 positive. Antibodies to CK1 and CK5 do not react with Paget cells, but react with normal epidermis.

Antibody to CK20 does not react with primary extramammary carcinoma of the vulva, i.e. those cases that are limited to vulva itself and have no other underlying malignancy. However, CK20 may react with tumor cells in perianal secondary extramammary carcinoma in which the cells of an underlying colorectal adenocarcinoma invade the epidermis. Rectal adenocarcinoma are positive for CK20 in 87% and coexpress CK7 in 22% cases (*Source:* Saad RS, et al. Appl Immunohistochem Mol Morphol. 2009;17:196-201).

Q.2 **The cervical lesion shown in Figure 7.2 will most likely be positive for which virus?**
   A. Human papilloma virus 6,11
   B. Human papilloma virus 16,18
   C. Human papilloma virus 31, 34
   D. Human papilloma virus 33, 35
   E. Human papilloma, multiple HPV subtypes

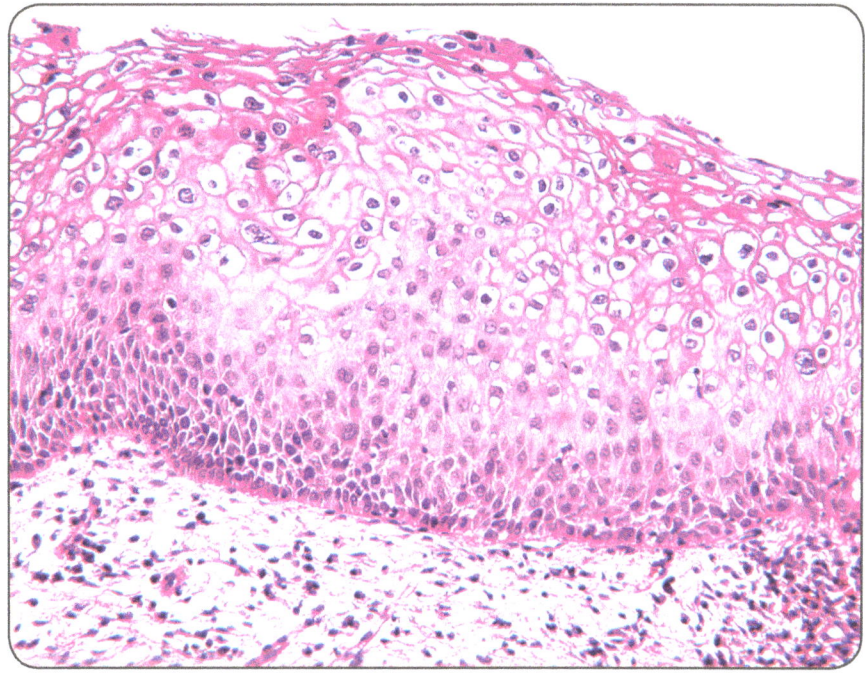

Figure 7.2

Answer: E. Human papilloma, multiple HPV subtypes

Comment: This low-grade squamous intraepithelial lesion (CIN1) with prominent koilocytosis is caused by human papilloma virus (HPV) but the subtype cannot be predicted from the histopathology of the lesion. In over one-half of cases, especially those with persistent lesions and those that progress to high-grade lesion there are **multiple HPV types** including both low risk and high risk viruses (*Source:* DeBrot L, et al. Cancer 2017; 125:138)

Q.3 **Which of the following is the best marker for endometrial stromal sarcoma?**
   A. Cytokeratin 7
   B. Wilms tumor 1 (WT 1)
   C. CD10
   D. c-KIT
   E. Inhibin

Answer: B. CD10

Comment: **CD10, a cell surface neutral endopeptidase** (originally recognized on the acute lymphoblastic leukemia cells and routinely used in hematopathology) is the best marker for endometrial stromal sarcoma and endometrial stromal nodules. However, the antibody to CD10 may react with some smooth muscle cells as well and accordingly, when applied to uterine tumors, it should be used only in a panel with other antibodies to smooth muscle cells. Antibody to CD10 reacts also with **clear cell renal carcinoma** including such rare renal tumors that have metastasized to the ovary or other parts of the female genital tract. Metastatic clear cell renal carcinomas must be distinguished from primary clear cell ovarian carcinomas, which are, however, CD10 negative.

Q.4 All the following cells or tumors express *p63, except:*
- **A.** Basal and parabasal cell of the normal cervical squamous epithelium
- **B.** Full thickness of epithelium in high grade intraepithelial cervical neoplasia
- **C.** Cervical squamous cell carcinoma
- **D.** Neuroendocrine carcinoma of cervix
- **E.** Vulvar Paget disease due to an underlying urothelial carcinoma

Answer: D. Neuroendocrine carcinoma of cervix

Comment: *p63* is expressed in the basal and parabasal cells of mature squamous epithelia of vulva, vagina and cervix. In high-grade CIN it is expressed throughout the entire thickness of the epithelium. It is also expressed in squamous cell and urothelial carcinoma, including the urothelial carcinoma of the bladder or urethra, which has spread to vulva in a pagetoid manner. p63 protein is not found in cervical neuroendocrine carcinomas.

Q.5 Which genetic change is most often encountered in atypical endometrial hyperplasia/EIN?
- **A.** Inactivating mutation or deletion of *PTEN* gene
- **B.** Activating mutation of *KRAS*
- **C.** *BRCA1* mutation
- **D.** *MLH1* inactivation
- **E.** *CTNNB1* (β-catenin gene) mutation

Answer: A. Inactivating mutation or a deletion of *PTEN* gene

Comment: The function of **all the genes** listed in this question has been found to be altered in atypical endometrial hyperplasia/EIN. The most common genetic change, paralleling the changes in endometrial carcinoma, is the inactivation of ***PTEN*** tumor suppressor gene. Changes in the function of other genes are found in not more than a quarter of all cases.

The inactivation of *PTEN* is found less commonly in atypical hyperplasia (less than 50% of all cases) than in endometrial endometrioid carcinoma (over 80% of all cases). These data indicate that *PTEN* gene product has an important role in histogenesis of endometrioid carcinoma, but also show that in itself the inactivation of *PTEN* gene seems not to be sufficient to produce endometrial malignancy. It has been postulated that some other genes must play an additive/synergistic role, and most evidence indicates that it could be most likely the *PAX2* gene.

***PAX2* gene** is inactivated in 70% cases of atypical endometrial hyperplasia. It has been recommended to use IHC antibodies to *PAX2* protein in combination with antibodies for *PTEN* protein. Such a combined approach gives positive results for both genes in about 30% cases; the specificity of this combined approach is high but its sensitivity is low. Furthermore, almost all leading authorities state that the routine **microscopic evaluation of biopsies** stained with H&E is still the best and most reliable approach to diagnosing atypical endometrial hyperplasia/EIN.

It should be noticed that *PAX2* and *PTEN* genes are inactivated in many cases of atypical hyperplasia/*EIN* and thus the gene product (protein) is not detectable in glands ("negative staining") in contrast to positive staining of normal glands. Staining for p53 and p16 gives also negative results in such lesions, albeit for different reasons.

Q.6 Immunohistochemical stains directed to one of the epitopes listed here will give positive results in essentially all cases of atypical endometrial hyperplasia/EIN. Which antigen is expressed on all cases of atypical endometrial hyperplasia/EIN?

    A. PAX2
    B. PTEN
    C. Estrogen receptor
    D. p53
    E. p16

Answer: C. Estrogen receptor

Comment: **Estrogen and progesterone receptors** are expressed on almost all cases of atypical endometrial hyperplasia/EIN. However, these biomarkers does not help in diagnosing the lesion or distinguishing it from endometrial carcinoma.

Q.7 Which of the following is found in most serous carcinoma of the endometrium and is useful for distinguishing it from endometrioid carcinoma?

    A. *TP53* mutation
    B. *PTEN* inactivation
    C. *KRAS* mutation
    D. Atypical endometrial hyperplasia/EIN present as precursor lesion
    E. Estrogen receptor found in more than 75% cases

Answer: A. *TP53* mutation

Comment: Serous carcinoma of endometrium is classified as type-2, non-endometrioid carcinoma. It shows *TP53* mutation in over 90% cases, in contrast to type-1 endometrioid carcinomas, which show *TP53* mutation in less than 10% cases. Serous carcinoma is not linked to hyperestrinism and prolonged or continuous estrogen stimulation.

PTEN inactivation and *KRAS* mutations are uncommonly found in serous carcinomas, and definitely less often than in endometrioid carcinomas. Estrogen receptors are expressed in only 20% of serous carcinoma, in contrast to endometrioid, which express both estrogen and progesterone receptors in 70–75% of cases. Serous carcinoma does not evolve from atypical endometrioid hyperplasia, which is a typical precursor lesion of endometrioid carcinoma.

Q.8 Distinguishing primary endocervical from endometrial endometrioid carcinoma may be difficult on curettage specimens, but it is important for therapeutic and prognostic purposes. Which of the following immunostain panels is most useful for distinguishing these two cancers?

    A. Desmin, inhibin, ER, PR
    B. p16, CEA, vimentin, ER
    C. Vimentin, AMACR, c-kit, Ki-67
    D. ER, PR, HER-2/neu
    E. CK7, CK20, TTF-1

Answer: B. p16, CEA, vimentin, ER

Comment: An immunohistochemical panel including **p16, carcinoembryonic antigen (CEA), vimentin, and estrogen receptor (ER)** is usually recommended for distinguishing primary endocervical from endometrial endometrioid carcinomas.

Endocervical carcinomas are diffusely positive for p16. CEA is positive in approximately 2/3 of all cases. Endometrial tumors are typically vimentin and ER positive, but CEA negative. p16 may be focally positive in endometrial carcinomas, but it does not show the strong, diffuse nuclear and cytoplasmic positivity as seen in endocervical adenocarcinomas.

Q.9 Mutation of which gene is most often detected in both the carcinomatous and sarcomatous component of endometrial carcinosarcomas?

A. *PTEN*
B. *p16*
C. *TP53*
D. *BRCA1*
E. *MLH-1*

Answer: **C. *TP53***

Comment: Several mutated genes may be detected in carcinosarcomas.

Mutated *TP53* is most often found genetic abnormality and it is the best evidence of the high-grade malignancy of these tumors.

PTEN mutation is common, and is taken as evidence of interconnectedness of carcinosarcoma and endometrioid carcinoma; these two tumors also share some epidemiological features, such as a link to hyperestrinism.

Gene *p16* (*CDKN2A*) is also commonly found in both carcinomatous and sarcomatous parts of endocervical carcinosarcomas.

Q.10 Which ovarian tumor reacts strongly with antibodies to CD117?

A. High-grade serous carcinoma
B. Brenner tumor
C. Granulosa cell tumor
D. Thecoma
E. Dysgerminoma

Answer: **E. Dysgerminoma**

Comment: **CD117 or c-KIT** is a transmembrane tyrosine kinase receptor, which is expressed in dysgerminomas. It is also expressed in gastrointestinal stromal tumors (GIST) which may spread on rare occasions to the female genital tract. Other tumors listed here do not react with antibodies to CD117.

Q.11 Which one of the following ovarian tumors reacts with antibodies to p63?

A. High-grade serous carcinoma
B. Brenner tumor
C. Granulosa cell tumor
D. Thecoma
E. Sclerosing stromal tumor

Answer: **B. Brenner tumor**

Comment: **Brenner tumors**, like transitional cell carcinomas of the urinary bladder react with antibodies to **p63**. Walthard nests are also positive.

Q.12 Tumor suppressor gene *PTEN* plays an important role in the pathogenesis of endometrioid carcinoma of the uterus. What is the name of the syndrome caused by the germline mutation of *PTEN* gene?

A. Gorlin syndrome
B. Cowden syndrome
C. Turner syndrome
D. Cronkhite-Canada syndrome
E. Peutz-Jeghers syndrome

Answer: B. Cowden syndrome

Comment: **Cowden syndrome** is associated with germline mutations of **PTEN** gene which makes the PTEN protein nonoperational in the mTOR signaling pathway. Cowden syndrome presents with macrocephaly, intestinal hamartomatous polyps, benign skin tumors (tricholemmomas), and acral keratoses. These patients also develop dysplastic gangliocytomas of cerebellum, and are at risk for developing carcinoma of the thyroid, endometrium, breast and ovaries.

Q.13 Translocation t(7;17)(p15;q21) resulting is *JAZF1-SUZ12* gene fusion gene is most often seen in which uterine tumor?

- A. Endometrioid carcinoma
- B. Low-grade endometrial stromal sarcoma
- C. High-grade endometrial stromal sarcoma
- D. PEComas
- E. Leiomyosarcomas

Answer: B. Low-grade endometrial stromal sarcoma

Comment: Translocation t(7;17)(p15;q21) resulting in **JAZF1-SUZ12 fusion gene** is seen in about 50% of **low-grade endometrial stromal sarcomas**. It is also found in most **endometrial stromal nodules.** This fusion gene is also known as *JAZF1/JJAZ1* gene fusion. Based on their structural features, these genes were given the acronyms *JAZF1*, for "juxtaposed with another zinc finger gene", and *JJAZ1*, for joined to *JAZF1* (lately named and referred in here as SUZ12 – "suppressor of zeste-12 protein") (*Source:* Hrzenjak A. Orphanet J. 2016;11:15).

Q.14 Translocation t(10,17)(q22;p13) resulting in the fusion gene *YWHAE-FAM22* is typically seen in which uterine tumor?

- A. Carcinosarcoma
- B. Low-grade endometrial stromal sarcoma
- C. High-grade endometrial stromal sarcoma
- D. PEComas
- E. Leiomyosarcoma

Answer: C. High-grade endometrial stromal sarcomas

Comment: Translocation t(10,17)(q22;p13) resulting in the fusion gene **YWHAE-FAM22** is typically seen in **high-grade endometrial stromal sarcomas.** It is not found in low grade ESS and endometrioid stromal nodules. *YWHAE* gene also known as 14-3-3ε, belongs to the family of **14-3-3 proteins**. It has multiple functions and regulates cytoskeletal configuration, metabolism, transcription, differentiation, and survival of eukaryotic cells. It is a highly conserved gene having the identical sequence in many species. By fusing with *FAM22*, a protein encoded by a gene in the NUT family, it forms a fusion gene that has oncogenic properties.

The presence of the fusion gene in high-grade tumors indicates that most of them evolve through a new set of genetic changes that are different from those in low-grade ESS or preneoplastic endometrial stromal cell lesions. There are however some high-grade ESS evolving from low-grade ESS and these contain microscopic foci of this low-grade tumor, which may also show the characteristic ESS cytogenetic changes such as the *JAZF1-SUZ12* fusion gene.

Q.15 MED12 is a subunit of the multiprotein complex mediator, an evolutionary-conserved regulator of transcription. *MED12* gene is most often mutated in which uterine tumor?

- A. Carcinosarcoma
- B. Leiomyoma
- C. High-grade endometrial stromal sarcoma

D. PEComa
E. Leiomyosarcoma

Answer: B. Leiomyoma

Comment: Oncogenic mutations of *MED12* occur in nearly 70% of uterine **leiomyomas.** Mutations of *MED12* are found in only a minority (15–18%) leiomyosarcomas of the uterus and are not found in extrauterine leiomyosarcomas (*Source:* Croce S, Chibon F. Eur J Cancer. 2015;51:1603-10). Tumors with *MED12* mutation do not show the translocation of genes for **non-histone proteins HMGA1 and HMGA1,** the second most common genetic change in uterine leiomyomas. Apparently, these genes act independently of one another and do not function in tandem in the pathogenesis of uterine leiomyomas (*Source:* Bertsch E, et al. Mod Pathol. 2014;27:1144-53).

Q.16 Germline mutation of the gene for fumarase is associated with an occurrence of which uterine tumor?
A. Endometrioid uterine carcinoma
B. Leiomyoma
C. Endometrial stromal sarcoma
D. PEComa
E. Leiomyosarcoma

Answer: B. Leiomyoma

Comment: Germline mutation of **fumarase gene** (**Reed syndrome**) is associated with a tendency for leiomyomatosis and **renal cell carcinoma**. Fumarase deficient leiomyomas may occur not only in the patients with Reed syndrome but also sporadically, accounting for approximately 1% of all uterine leiomyomas (*Source:* Miettinen M, et al. Am J Surg Pathol. 2016; 40:1661-9).

Q.17 Inactivation of *TSC2* gene with activation of the mammalian target of ripamycin (mTOR) is a constant feature of which uterine tumor?
A. Endometrioid uterine carcinoma
B. Leiomyoma
C. Endometrial stromal sarcoma
D. PEComa
E. Leiomyosarcoma

Answer: D. PEComa

Comment: **TSC2 (tuberous sclerosis) gene** encoding the protein **tuberin** is inactivated in most perivascular epithelioid cell tumors (PEComas), including those found in the uterus. Germline inactivation of *TSC2* gene is found in tuberous sclerosis, a condition marked by an increased incidence of PEComas. However, **sporadic uterine PEComas** also show inactivation of this gene.

Q.18 The infundibular part of the fallopian tube contained microscopic foci of multilayered epithelium composed of atypical secretory cells showing a high nucleus/cytoplasmic ratio and no polarity. The MIB-1 proliferative index was 70%. Antibody to which antigen will selectively react with these cells?
A. PAX 2
B. PAX8
C. p53
D. p16
E. ALDH1

Answer: C. p53

Comment: The foci of multilayered epithelium composed of atypical non-polarized non-ciliated (secretory) cells showing a high nucleus/cytoplasmic and an increased MIB-1 proliferative index (over 50%) are classified as **serous tubal intraepithelial carcinoma (STIC).** Foci of STIC react strongly with the antibody to **p53** and are considered to be potential precursors of high-grade serous carcinoma of the ovary. STIC may react with antibody to p16, but it also reacts with benign epithelial hyperplasia and is thus not useful. Antibodies to WT1 and PAX8 also give positive results, but they react with non-neoplastic epithelium as well. PAX2 and ALDH1 are actually lost in STIC.

Aldehyde dehydrogenase1 (ALDH1) is preferentially expressed in endometrioid carcinomas of the ovary and could be a marker indicative of better clinical outcome of ovarian tumors (*Source:* Chang B, et al. Mod Pathol. 2009; 22:817-23).

Q.19 Which germline mutation is most often identified in women with primary carcinoma of the fallopian tubes?

- A. *BRCA1* and *BRCA2*
- B. *MHL-1*
- C. *TP53*
- D. p16
- E. *WT-1*

Answer: **A.** *BRCA1* and *BRCA2*

Comment: ***BRCA1* and *BRCA2*** mutations are found in one-third of all women with primary fallopian tube carcinomas. Heterozygous germline mutations of these genes are found in approximately 1:400 women in the Western world, and 1:40 of women of Ashkenazy Jewish descent. For those women there is an increased lifetime risk of fimbrial tubal/ovarian cancer, which has been estimated to be 40% for *BRCA1* and 10% for *BRCA2* positive women. Risk reducing salpingo-oophorectomy will reduce the risk by 80–90%, but will not eliminate it entirely.

Q.20 Inactivation of which tumor suppressor gene plays a role in the early pathogenesis of ovarian endometrioid adenocarcinoma?

- A. *BRCA1*
- B. *BRCA2*
- C. *PTEN*
- D. *WT-1*
- E. *NF-1*

Answer: **C.** *PTEN*

Comment: ***PTEN* gene** which encodes the phosphatase and tensin protein serves as a tumor suppressor gene and its inactivation or loss is found in a significant number of stage I endometrioid carcinomas. This fact coupled with the finding of *PTEN* inactivation in foci of endometriosis adjacent to the ovarian carcinoma, suggests that this gene plays an important role in the pathogenesis of endometrioid carcinoma of the ovary. Likewise *PTEN* is instrumental in the pathogenesis of endometrial adenocarcinoma of the uterus, further supporting the view that the endometrial and the ovarian endometrioid carcinomas are closely related tumors. Current immunohistochemical methods for demonstrating *PTEN*, however, are not reliable enough to justify routine diagnostic use of this marker.

Q.21 In contrast to high-grade serous carcinoma (HGSC), endometrioid carcinoma of the ovary is unreactive with antibody to which antigen?

- A. Cytokeratin 7 (CK7)
- B. Vimentin
- C. Estrogen receptor
- D. Progesterone receptor
- E. p53

Answer: E. p53

Comment: **Endometrioid carcinoma** of the ovary does not react with antibodies to **p53** and **WT 1**, two antibodies that usually react with HGSC. All other antibodies typically react with endometrioid carcinoma cells.

Q.22 All the following antibodies react with mesothelioma but are nonreactive with high-grade serous carcinoma of the ovary, *except:*

   A. Anti-cytokeratin CK5/6
   B. Anti-podoplanin (D2-40)
   C. Anti-calretinin
   D. Thrombomodulin
   E. MOC31

Answer: E. MOC31

Comment: **Antibody MOC31** reacts with **adenocarcinomas** but does not react with **mesothelioma**. All other antibodies are good markers for mesothelioma. When trying to distinguish mesothelioma from ovarian adenocarcinoma it is best to combine two antibodies to adenocarcinoma related glycoproteins (like Ber-EP4 and MOC31) with two mesothelioma reactive antibodies such as those recognizing calretinin, or podoplanin (D2.40).

Q.23 Figure 7.3 shows an ovarian tumor carrying a mutation of *SMARC4*, a gene encoding a protein in the catalytic unit of the *SWI/SSNF* chromatin remodeling complex. What is the most likely diagnosis?

   A. Small cell undifferentiated carcinoma, hypercalcemic type
   B. Small cell carcinoma, pulmonary type
   C. Small cell carcinoma, nonpulmonary type
   D. Transitional-like carcinoma
   E. High-grade serous carcinoma

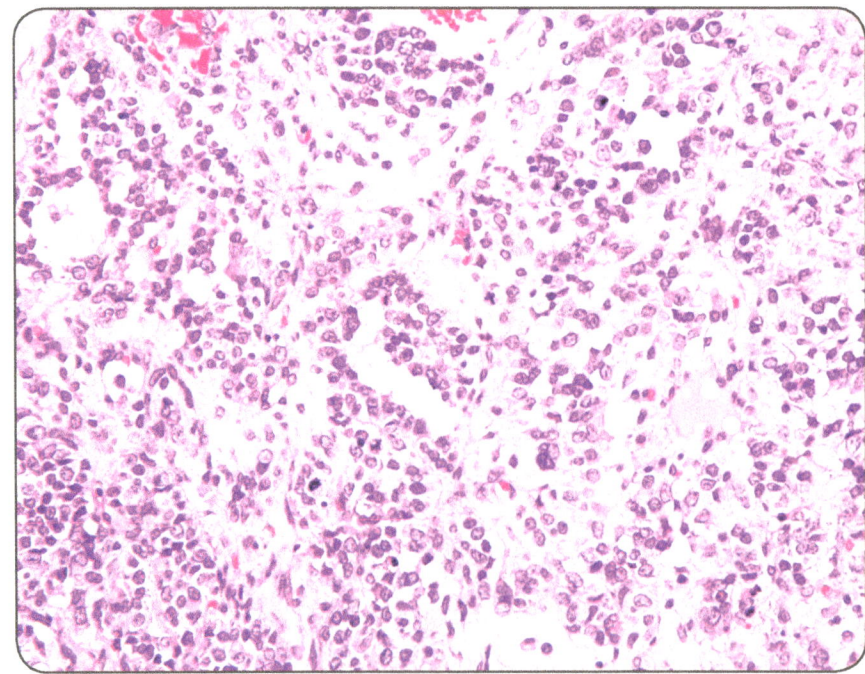

Figure 7.3

Answer: A. Small cell undifferentiated carcinoma, hypercalcemic type

Comment: Mutation of *SMARC4* (SWI/SNF related, matrix associated, actin dependent regulator of chromatin, subfamily a, member 4) has been found in all small **cell undifferentiated carcinoma, hypercalcemic type,** and is considered to be a molecular signature of this malignancy (*Source:* Jelinic P, et al. Mod Pathol. 2016;29:60-6).

Q.24 Which gene plays an important role in the pathogenesis of ovarian granulosa cell tumors?
- A. *VHL*
- B. *FOXL2*
- C. *PTEN*
- D. *MHL-1*
- E. *PTCH*

Answer: B. *FOXL2*

Comment: Protein **FOXL2**, a forkhead transcription factor with a DNA binding domain, plays a critical role in the **development of the ovary**. Missense point mutations of *FOXL2* gene encoding this protein are found in almost all **adult granulosa cell tumors.** This is taken as evidence for the pathogenic role of the mutated gene in the histogenesis of adult granulosa cell tumors. The mutated *FOXL2* gene can be demonstrated by IHC in the nuclei of tumor cells.

Q.25 Trisomy 12 and 14 and monosomy 22 can be demonstrated by FISH in the sex cord stromal tumor shown in Figure 7.4. What is the most likely diagnosis?
- A. Adult granulosa cell tumor
- B. Juvenile granulosa cell tumor
- C. Fibroma
- D. Thecoma
- E. Steroid cell tumor

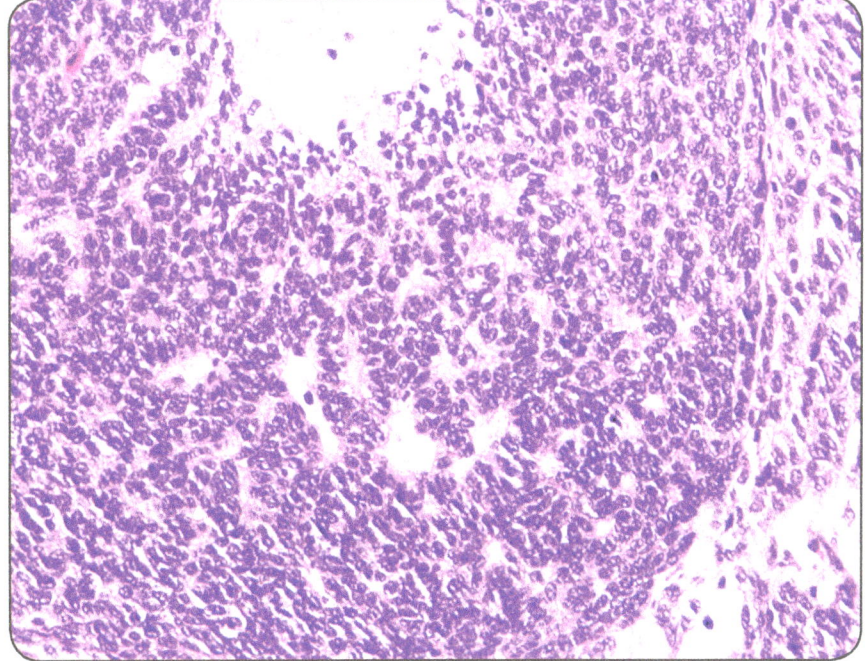

Figure 7.4

Answer: A. Adult granulosa cell tumor

Comment: Trisomy 12 and 14 and monosomy 22 can be demonstrated by FISH in **adult granulosa cell tumors** and their metastases.

Q.26 Which ovarian tumor is found in patients who have germline mutation of the tumor suppressor gene *STK11* (also known as *LKB1*)?

    A. Adult granulosa cell tumors
    B. Juvenile granulosa cell tumor
    C. Sex cord tumor with annular tubules
    D. Sertoli-Leydig cell tumor
    E. Sclerosing stromal tumor

Answer: C. Sex cord tumor with annular tubules

Comment: Mutations of the **STK11 tumor suppressor gene** (also known as *LKB1*) are the cause of most cases of **Peutz-Jeghers syndrome**. Patients with this syndrome often have ovarian **sex cord tumors with annular tubules (SCTAT)**.

Q.27 All the following genes have been found to play a pathogenetic role in ovarian sex cord-stromal tumors, *except:*

    A. *FOXL2*
    B. *STK11*
    C. *DICER1*
    D. *CTNNB1*
    E. *PTEN*

Answer: E. *PTEN*

Comment: **FOXL2** (forkhead transcription factor) is mutated in over 90% of all adult granulosa cell tumors.
    STK11 (serine threonine kinase, also known as liver kinase B1, LKB) undergoes germline mutations, which act as a tumor suppressor gene in patients with Peutz-Jeghers syndrome and **ovarian SCTAT**.
    DICER1 (a gene encoding a double stranded ribonuclease) is mutated in over 60% of **Sertoli-Leydig cell tumors**, especially those that secrete male sex hormones. *DICER1* mutation may link the rare concurrence of SLC tumors of the ovary and thyroid tumors (*Source:* Durieux E, et al. Virchows Arch. 2016;468: 631-6).
    CTNNB1 (beta-catenin gene) is found to be involved in the rare **microcystic stromal tumor** (*Source:* Kopczynski J, et al. Appl Immunohistochem Mol Morphol. 2016; 24:e28-e33).
    PTEN gene is not involved in the pathogenesis of sex cord-stromal tumors but plays a role in the pathogenesis of endometrioid adenocarcinomas of the uterus and ovary.

Q.28 Antibodies to which antigen react with the nuclei of dysgerminoma and embryonal carcinoma?

    A. Placental alkaline phosphatase (PLAP)
    B. c-KIT (CD117)
    C. Podoplanin (D2-40)
    D. SALL4
    E. Cytokeratin CK7

Answer: D. SALL4

Comment: **SALL4 is** a good marker for undifferentiated tumors cells of all **germ cell tumors** including dysgerminoma, embryonal carcinoma, yolk sac carcinoma, and gonadoblastoma. SALL4 (acronym which stands for Sal-like protein 4) is a transcription factor encoded by a gene from the Spalt-*like* (*SALL*) gene family, and is also known as a key embryonic stem cells factor.

Q.29 Gonadoblastoma occurs in phenotypic females whose karyotype has which one of the following chromosomal changes?

- A. Two X chromosomes
- B. One X chromosome
- C. Chromosomal mosaicism with fragments of Y chromosome
- D. None of the above
- E. All the above

Answer: **C. Chromosomal mosaicism with fragments of Y chromosome**

Comment: Some genes on the **Y chromosome** play an important role in the pathogenesis of **gonadoblastomas,** most of which arise in dysgenetic gonads. The gonadoblastoma locus on the human Y chromosome (GBY) is postulated to serve normal functions in spermatogenesis, but could become oncogenic. The **testis-specific protein Y-linked (TSPY)** found in all so far tested gonadoblastomas is the putative gene involved in their pathogenesis (*Source:* Lau YF, et al. Syst Biol Reprod Med. 2011;57:22-34).

Q.30 Which malignant tumor develops most often in women with Cowden syndrome?

- A. Breast carcinoma
- B. Vulvar carcinoma
- C. Endocervical carcinoma
- D. Endometrial carcinoma
- E. Ovarian carcinoma

Answer: **A. Breast carcinoma**

Comment: Life time risk of breast carcinoma in Cowden syndrome is 85%. The risk for endometrial adenocarcinoma is 28%. (Eng C, 2016; search WWW using the term "PTEN hamartoma syndromes").

Q.31 Programmed cell death 1/programmed cell death ligand (PD-1/PD-L1) is expressed in cells of which ovarian tumor?

- A. Sertoli-Leydig cell tumor
- B. Thecoma
- C. Teratoma
- D. Choriocarcinoma
- E. Granulosa cell tumor

Answer: **D. Choriocarcinoma**

Comment: **Programmed cell death 1/programmed cell death ligand (PD-1/PD-L1)** is expressed in **choriocarcinoma** or trophoblastic cells of mixed germ cell tumors. PD-L1 immunohistochemical staining is considered a potential predictor of clinical response to PD-1/PD-L1 immune checkpoint inhibitor treatment (*Source:* Inaguma S, et al. Am J Surg Pathol. 2016; 40:1133-42). PD-L1 is also expressed on the trophoblasts of the normal placenta.

Q.32 A mutation of which gene is responsible for the majority of hereditary breast cancers?
   A. *BRCA2*
   B. *BRCA1*
   C. *TP53*
   D. *PTEN*
   E. *CDH1*

Answer: B. *BRCA1*

Comment: **BRCA1 gene mutations** are responsible for the majority of hereditary breast cancers followed by *BRCA2* gene mutations. These two genes are responsible for 80–90% of all hereditary cancers of breast and ovary. Germline mutations of other genes may also be associated with breast cancer but are uncommon. Thus, *TP53* plays role in Li-Fraumeni syndrome, *PTEN* in Cowden syndrome, *CDH1* in diffuse gastric and lobular breast cancer.

Q.33 Which of the following genes is most often mutated in hereditary cancer syndromes associated with development of breast carcinoma in men?
   A. *TP53*
   B. *BRCA1*
   C. *BRCA2*
   D. *PTEN*
   E. *CHEK2*

Answer: C. *BRCA2*

Comment: Most familial male **breast cancers** are associated with mutations of **BRCA2**, rather than *BRCA1* gene. Mutations of *TP53* (Li-Fraumeni syndrome), *PTEN* (Cowden syndrome), and *CHEK2* mutation-associated cancer syndrome predispose to development of breast cancer in women. Clinical and pathologic features of male breast cancer associated with *BRCA2* mutation do not differ from those in sporadic male breast cancers. As a group male breast carcinomas appear to be more frequently ER, PR, and androgen receptor positive and Her2/neu negative than female breast carcinomas.

Q.34 Which of the following is the most common somatic gene mutation in breast cancer?
   A. *BRCA1*
   B. *PIK3CA*
   C. *PTEN*
   D. *TP53*
   E. *Her2*

Answer: D. *TP53*

Comment: **TP53 gene mutations** are the most common somatic mutations across all cancer subtypes including breast cancer. These are particularly common in Her2-positive and triple-negative breast cancers.

Inherited *TP53* gene mutations cause Li–Fraumeni syndrome.

PIK3CA and **PTEN** gene mutations are also common and these genetic alterations cause deregulation of mTOR signaling pathway.

BRCA1 mutations are typically seen in triple-negative breast carcinomas and in a subset of familial breast cancers.

Her2 gene mutations (in contrast to *Her2* gene amplification) are rare but have been increasingly reported in various cancers including breast cancer.

Q.35 *Her2/neu* **gene amplification by in situ hybridization method (a single-probe system) is defined as:**

- A. >4 signals per cell nucleus (on average)
- B. >10 signals per cell nucleus (on average)
- C. >6 signals per cell nucleus (on average)
- D. >8 signals per cell nucleus (on average)
- E. >12 signals per cell nucleus (on average)

Answer: C. >6 signals per cell nucleus (on average)

Comment: In situ hybridization methods (e.g. FISH and CISH) are routinely employed for the evaluation of *Her2/neu* gene amplification in breast cancer. When a single-probe system is used, the tumor is considered amplified for *Her2/neu* if >6 signals per cell nucleus are observed (on average). For dual probes *Her2/neu*: *CEP17* ratio should be ≥2 (on average) (ASCO/CAP recommendation 2013).

Q.36 Figure 7.5 shows the results of a chromogenic in situ hybridization (CISH) assay. How are these results best interpreted?

- A. Normal *Her2/CEP17* ratio (non-amplified Her2) (<2)
- B. Increased *Her2/CEP17* ratio (amplification) (>2)
- C. Increased *CEP17* copy number (polysomy)
- D. Decreased *Her2* copy number (<2)

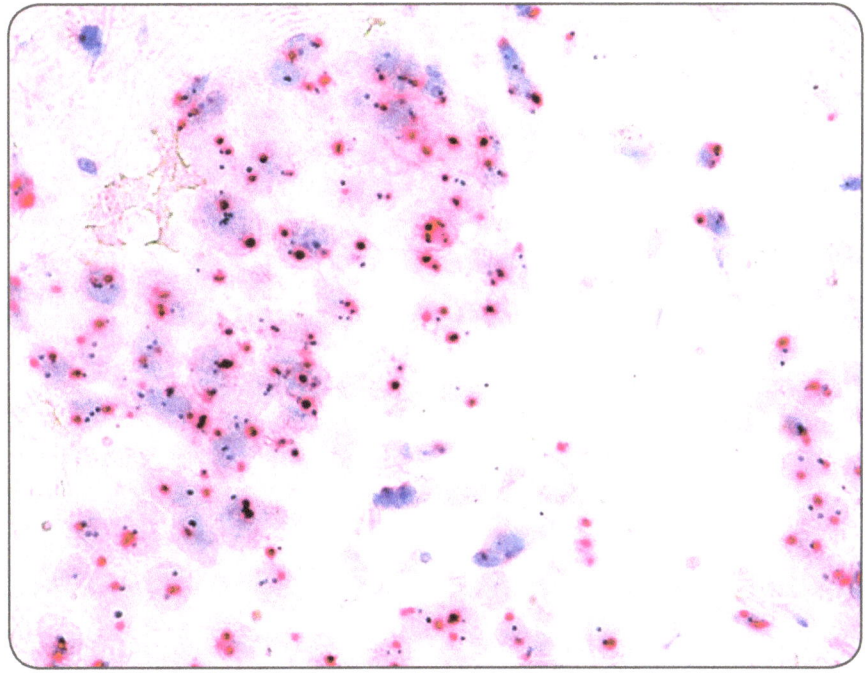

Figure 7.5

Answer: A. Normal *Her2/CEP17* ratio (non-amplified Her2) (<2).

Comment: The Figure shows a dual chromogenic in situ hybridization assay with *Her2/CEP17* ratio <2, implying no *Her2* gene amplification. Polysomy is usually defined as ≥3 *CEP17* copies per cell.

Q.37 Which of the following statements regarding OncotypeDX (Genomic Health, Inc.) is correct?
- A. It predicts a chemotherapy benefit in ER-negative, node-negative breast cancer
- B. It predicts a hormonal therapy benefit in ER-positive, node-negative breast cancer
- C. It predicts a hormonal therapy benefit in ER-positive, node-positive breast cancer
- D. It predicts a chemotherapy benefit in ER-positive, node-negative breast cancer

Answer: D. It predicts a chemotherapy benefit in ER-positive, node-negative breast cancer

Comment: OncotypeDX is an **RT-PCR-based assay** that analyzes 21 genes (16 cancer-associated + 5 reference genes) to provide a recurrence score as an indicator of patient's outcome. Although, it has been shown to provide valuable information in both node-positive and node-negative, ER-positive breast cancers treated with endocrine (hormonal) therapy, it is primarily used in selected patients with ER-positive, node-negative breast cancer to predict a chemotherapy benefit.

Q.38 The 70-gene signature test has been developed to provide:
- A. Predictive information in patients with early breast cancer
- B. Prognostic information in patients with early breast cancer
- C. Predictive information in patients with advanced breast cancer
- D. Prognostic information in patients with advanced breast cancer

Answer: B. Prognostic information in patients with early breast cancer

Comment: 70-gene signature is a microarray-based assay aimed to provide the prognostic information for patients with early breast cancer (stages pT1-2). The test is dichotomous and classifies the tumors into "good" and "bad" prognosis. The clinical utility of this assay is supported by the level II of evidence.

Q.39 Recurrent chromosomal translocation t (6;9) (q22-23; p23-24) is a feature of which breast carcinoma?
- A. Mucoepidermoid carcinoma
- B. Adenoid cystic carcinoma
- C. Polymorphous carcinoma
- D. Adenomyoepithelioma
- E. Secretory carcinoma

Answer: B. Adenoid cystic carcinoma

Comment: **Recurrent chromosomal translocation t(6;9)(q22-23;p23-24)** resulting in fusion transcripts of *MYB* and *NFIB* genes is a feature of mammary **adenoid cystic carcinoma** (ACC). Identical genetic alteration is present in its counterpart affecting salivary glands. This genetic alteration is not present in other mammary neoplasms mentioned above.

Q.40 A loss of 16q chromosome is a feature of which type of breast cancer?
- A. Lobular carcinoma
- B. Metaplastic carcinoma
- C. Medullary carcinoma
- D. Micropapillary carcinoma
- E. Secretory carcinoma

Answer: A. Lobular carcinoma

Comment: A **loss of 16q chromosome** is characteristically seen in **lobular carcinoma** affecting ***CDH1*** gene which encodes E-cadherin, a cell adhesion protein typically lost in lobular carcinoma. A subset of low-grade ductal carcinomas may also lose 16q, but the targeted genes are yet to be determined. In contrast, all the above mentioned subtypes (b-d) are high-grade carcinomas, which rarely exhibit deletions at 16q. Secretory carcinoma is a rare subtype with triple-negative phenotype and recurrent t(12;15) translocation (*ETV6-NTRK3*).

Q.41 Next-generation sequencing assay is aimed to detect all the following, *except:*

   A. Mutations
   B. Copy number variations
   C. DNA rearrangements
   D. Protein expression
   E. RNA-editing

Answer: **D. Protein expression**

Comment: **Next-generation sequencing assay** (NGS) is a new, promising, high-throughput technique, which may sequence thousands or millions of sequences in one reaction. It is a DNA/RNA-based assay that has revolutionized cancer genomics and profiling. NGS can **sequence entire genome** (all DNA), **exome** (coding gene regions), to explore gene **mutations, rearrangements, amplifications,** or **deletions** and **transcriptome** (RNA) to analyze gene expression levels, splicing variants, and **RNA editing**.

Q.42 What are the best immunohistochemical stains for distinguishing low-grade squamous intraepithelial (LSIL) lesions from high-grade squamous intraepithelial (HSIL) lesions of the cervix?

   A. Inhibin and desmin
   B. Vimentin and cytokeratin CK7
   C. CK5/6 and p63
   D. p16 and Ki-67
   E. Estrogen and progesterone receptors

Answer: **D. p16 and Ki-67**

Comment: **p16** is widely used as an immunohistochemical surrogate marker for high-risk human papillomavirus (HPV), such as, HPV-16 and HPV-18. In **LSIL**, the p16 expression may be confined to the lower one-third or one-half of the squamous epithelium or show only focal immunoreactivity. In **HSIL** p16 immunoexpression usually involves two-third or full thickness of the squamous epithelium. Ki-67 may show increased positivity both in neoplastic and reactive conditions, but it is more prominent and involves the entire epithelium in HSIL. Ki-67 immunohistochemistry should be used in combination with p16.

Inhibin is mostly used in the differential diagnostic work up of ovarian sex cord-stromal tumors. Desmin is used to confirm the myogenic differentiation of a tumor. Antibodies to vimentin and cytokeratin CK7 are not useful in this case.

Bibliography

1. Clement PB, Young RH. Atlas of gynecologic surgical pathology. 3rd edition. Saunders, Elsevier: Philadelphia; 2013
2. Crum CP, Quick CM, Laury AR, Peters WA, Hirsch MS. Gynecologic and obstetric pathology. Elsevier: Philadelphia; 2015.
3. Hicks DG, Lester SC. Diagnostic pathology breast, 2nd edition. Elsevier: Philadelphia; 2016.
4. Hoda SA, Brogi E, Koerner FC, Rosen PP (Eds). Rosen's breast pathology, 4th edition. Wolters Kluwer: Philadelphia; 2014.
5. Kurman RJ, Ellenson LH, Ronnett BM (Eds). Blaustein's pathology of the female genital tract. 6th edition. Springer: New York; 2011.
6. Kurman RJ, Carcangiu ML, Herrington CS, Young RH (Eds). WHO classification of tumours of the female reproductive organs. 4th edition. IARC: Lyon; 2015.
7. Lakhani SR, Ellis IO, Schnitt SJ, Tan PH, vam de Vijver MJ (Eds). WHO classification of tumours of the breast. 4th edition. IARC: Lyon; 2012.
8. Mutter GL, Prat J (Eds). Pathology of the female reproductive tract. 3rd edition. Churchill Livingstone, Elsevier: Edinburgh; 2014.
9. Nucci MR, Oliva E (Eds). Gynecologic pathology. Churchill Livingstone, Elsevier: Edinburgh; 2009.
10. Nucci MR, Oliva E (Eds). Diagnostic pathology: Gynecological. Amyrsis; 2015.
11. O'Malley FP, Pinder SE, Mulligan AM, Goldblum JR (Eds). Breast pathology, 2nd Edition. Saunders Elsevier: Philadelphia; 2011.
12. Prat J. Pathology of the ovary. Saunders, Elsevier: Philadelphia; 2004.
13. Robboy SJ, Mutter GL, Prat J, Bentley RC, Russell P, Anderson MC. Robboy's pathology of the female reproductive tract. 2nd Edition. Saunders, Elsevier: Philadelphia; 2009.
14. Schnitt SJ, Colins LC. Biopsy interpretation of the breast. 2nd edition. Wolters Kluwer: Lippincott Williams and Wilkins; 2013.
15. Wick M, LiVolsi VA, Pfeifer JD, Stelow EB, Wakely PE, Jr. (Eds). Silverberg's principles and practice of surgical pathology and cytopathology. Volume 1. 5th edition. Cambridge University Press; 2015.

www.ingramcontent.com/pod-product-compliance
Lightning Source LLC
Chambersburg PA
CBHW040539220526
45473CB00016B/2979